AN ENCYCLOPEDIA OF HOMOEOPATHY

A survey of the homoeopathic method and approach in alphabetical form including:- the history, philosophy, major personalities, remedies and illnesses. Written by a doctor with over 30 years experience of holistic medicine.

By the same author:-

Homoeopathic Medicine

The Homoeopathic Treatment of Emotional Illness

A Woman's Guide to Homoeopathy

Understanding Homoeopathy

Talking About Homoeopathy

An Encyclopedia of Homoeopathy

The Principles, Art and Practice of Homoeopathy

Emotional Health

Personal Growth and Creativity

The Side-Effects Book

Homoeopathy for Pregnancy and Nursing Mothers

Homoeopathy for Babies and Children

Homoeopathy for Everyday Stress Problems

Homoeopathy for Teenager Problems

Homoeopathy for the Menopause

AN ENCYCLOPEDIA OF HOMOEOPATHY

A comprehensive reference book and survey of homoeopathy from its beginnings to the present day

by

Dr Trevor Smith
MA, MB, BChir, DPM, MFHom

INSIGHT

Insight Editions
Worthing, Sussex
England

WARNING

The contents of this volume are for general interest only and individual persons should always consult their medical adviser about a particular problem or before stopping or changing an existing treatment.

First published 1983
New 2nd edition 1994

Published by Insight Editions
Worthing
Sussex
England

British Library Cataloguing in Publication Data
A catalogue record for this book is available from the British Library.

ISBN

0-496670 21 8 (Hard Back)
0 946670 22 6 (Soft Back)

Cover photograph by the author.

PREFACE

Aims and Objectives

The encyclopedia clarifies and explains the following major areas of Homoeopathic interest.

1) The most important historical personalities and prescribers of the homoeopathic scene of the last 150 years.

2) The common illnesses in outline with a brief list of their relevant remedies.

3) The major remedies, with a description of their action.

4) The essential areas of homoeopathic philosophy (involving the approach and the process of prescribing) are dealt with and contrasted with the conventional allopathic approach to the patient and his illness.

ACKNOWLEDGMENTS

The following friends and colleagues contributed generously of their time and expertise to ensure that the text is as accurate and up-to-date as possible.

John Alman, John Ainsworth, Dr Hamish Boyd,
Cheryl A. Gill, Mary Gooch, Dr Richard Savage,
Jan Sherrington, Julian Winston.

This book is dedicated with gratitude to the many patients who have worked patiently with me - accepting my limitations with as much spirit and grace as my more inspired moments. Their understanding, humour and faith has been an example and source of strength over the past 35 years.

Introduction

All cure is from within; medicines themselves do not cure - not even the homoeopathic ones. They only act nby deeply mobilising the individual pathways of vital reaction towards cure. What man has caused - in illness and disease - man can also cure. Often the causative factor lies within the mind, undermining resistance and vitality. This vital reaction - really a movement of energy within the person - is in us all, provided it can be mobilised. Homoeopathy is one of the most important and effective tools to stimulate a curative response because it acts like a natural catalyst. Only in recent years has the inherent power of the remedies become more recognised by the public.

However more doctors need to know and to appreciate homoeopathy. This is a slow process, because medical education is still rooted in the synthetic and pharmaceutical approach of suppression of symptoms, so that homoeopathy often appears quite alien, unscientific and suspect.

Homoeopathy does not promise or guarantee that a cure will occur, but it does promise a method of individual approach and treatment. It has genuine potential for cure, provided that the method is not contraindicated, or a conventional approach for a particular physical or mechanical problem more indicated and superior.

Homoeopathy is holistic and offers what is best for the individual with an overall caring attitude. An unbiased approach is essential where the patient comes first and not the principles of any method or the need to prescribe.

Homoeopathy is a unique system of medicine with a wide range of potential and treatments. Many of its therapeutic resources have not yet been fully recognized nor its benefits to the patient when prescribed in proper depth and potency. The method should not be abused by implying that it is indicated where other methods are better advised and of more value.

There is more to homoeopathy than just matching the symptom-picture of the patient to the toxic proving profile of the remedy. The Law of Similars is a fundamental guideline to prescribing, but the experienced practitioner must also take the potency into account. The more recent high serial dilutions offer a greater dimension to homoeopathic thinking because in this form they are able to mobilise the more inflexible and defended parts of both mind and body.

Because of its action on temperament and attitudes as well as the physical, homoeopathy opens avenues of therapeutic possibility previously thought impossible.

For the best results it is not sufficient to just guess at the correct potency or to prescribe by rule-of-thumb. A proper assessment must be made during the initial diagnostic consultation of the true level of primary disturbance. This should be discussed with the patient during the consultation-dialogue and then mobilised by the correct prescription.

The potency determines the depth reached by the remedy and this should be regularly re-appraised. The correct remedy may be the constitutional one or it may be a 'low' dilution, more pathological one, but whenever a 'high' potency is chosen for whatever reason it should always be followed by a back-up consultation in about 2 weeks to provide essential support for the patient. At that time it may not be necessary to re-prescribe because improvement has occurred. But where change or mobilisation gives rise to anxiety, there will be a need for extra reassurance and possibly a further remedy. This is the essence of good prescribing.

Homoeopathy should not be a last resort, but prescribed early and where indicated. It is hoped that this volume will provide a small contribution to the field of therapeutics and a better appreciation of the method and its potential.

7 Upper Harley Street
London NW1 4PS

ADVICE ON TAKING HOMOEOPATHIC REMEDIES

Sources of remedies

The remedies recommended throughout the book should be purchased directly from a homoeopathic pharmacy or health shop. Always ensure that your remedies are from a reliable source and take them in the sixth centesimal or 6c potency.

Using the remedies

The potencies or strengths, come as small round pills or tablets, made of sucrose (or lactose). If you are sensitive to lactose, you should order your remedies directly from a homoeopathic pharmacy, requesting a pure sucrose or lactose-free pill base for the remedies. Because the medicine, or homoeopathic dilution is applied directly to the surface of the pill, they should not be handled. They are best placed directly into the mouth from the lid of the container and sucked under the tongue. They should always be taken at least 20 minutes before or after food or drink (except water), orthodox medicines, vitamin or mineral supplements and toothpaste.

Substances to avoid

Do not drink peppermint tea when taking homoeopathic remedies. Avoid coffee, tea and cocoa, because their high caffeine content may diminish their effect.

Keeping the remedies fresh and active

The medicines should be stored in a cool, dry, dark area, away from strong odours, especially camphor, oil of wintergreen, perfume, essential oils, after-shave and soap. In this way, their action will last indefinitely.

Diet and alcohol

A bland diet is recommended, not eating to excess, or using strong spices. Alcohol should be avoided, and smoking reduced or stopped altogether during treatment, especially for lung, heart, or circulatory problems.

How long should remedies be taken for

Remedies should be taken for as long as any symptoms persist - and then stopped. If new symptoms arise during homoeopathic treatment, they should be watched carefully, especially if they have occurred in the past. The homoeopathic action may sometimes cause earlier symptoms to reappear. They are usually fleeting, but if persistent, they will require a new remedy.

Aggravation of symptoms

An aggravation of symptoms, after taking the remedies, is a positive sign and means the potencies are working well. It is usually short-lived, and does not undermine the overall sense of well-being and improved vitality.

Side-effects

If you use them correctly, there are no side-effects or risks from homoeopathy. If you take a wrong remedy, or a whole box of the pills, they will cause no harm. The remedies can be safely used during pregnancy, breast feeding, or given to the youngest baby. It is unwise to continue taking a homoeopathic remedy after the symptoms have been relieved.

Homoeopathy and orthodox medicines
The remedies do not interact with orthodox medicines, or undermine their action. If you are given a course of antibiotics, it is best to stop homoeopathic remedies for this period. Some orthodox drugs, especially steroids, may reduce or neutralise the homoeopathic effect.

Pain
Homoeopathy will help with some types of pain and spasm, but it is not the treatment of choice for very acute or severe pain and if this occurs, orthodox treatment is recommended.

Homoeopathy and the age of the patient
Homoeopathy acts at every age, the reaction varying with age, strength, and the intrinsic resistance or vital energy reserves of the patient. It acts very quickly in a child, or fit young person, but is much slower in an elderly person, particularly if old, weak, or feeble.

Homoeopathy and acute illness of the elderly
It is often better initially, to give an orthodox treatment to an elderly person during an acute illness. If possible, use homoeopathy when convalescent, and before severe weakness occurs.

Safety of the homoeopathic approach
Homoeopathy is nevertheless helpful in the older age group for:- muddled thinking, poor memory, insomnia, restlessness, anxiety or tension problems. It does not cause confusion of the mind or agitation, which may be a severe problem when some orthodox drugs are used.

A

Abrasions and Cuts

Clean the wound with *Calendula* cream or tincture. If the patient is shocked with bruising, give *Arnica* 30c hourly until there is improvement. If there is shock with agitation and fear shown, give *Aconitum* 30c every 15 minutes until free from shock. Where the wound is dirty give *Hepar sulph* or *Mercurius.* For a penetrating wound give *Ledum* 6c or *Hypericum* 6c. When there is a foreign body, or the remnants of it in the wound, this must be removed immediately - either by the family or the nearest hospital casualty department.

Abscess

This is a painful inflammatory condition of the skin or other internal organ where there is swelling with heat, redness and pulsating pain causing restlessness and discomfort. In severe cases the abscess may become toxic, provoking drowsiness and fever, with a discharge of pus.
REMEDIES
Anthracinum, Belladonna, Hepar sulph, Mercurius, Silicea, Sulphur.

Accidents

When there is damage to tissues caused by trauma. Often these are the common first-aid conditions which occur in the home. *Arnica* is always the most important immediate remedy for shock. Any bleeding must be stopped by local pressure. Where there has been a severe burn or scald give Rescue Remedy 5 drops every hour with *Arnica* 30c in a single dose daily until recovery occurs. Give *Cantharis* 6 for burning discomfort, *Urtica urens* where there is discomfort from swelling and fluid retention. If the condition is severe the patient must be urgently hospitalised in a specialised burns unit.

Accident-Proneness

The tendency to be frequently involved in one form of accident or another, for underlying psychological reasons.

REMEDIES

Baryta carb. when associated with the elderly.

Kali carb. when due to undue nervousness.

Lycopodium the person is always distracted or preoccupied elsewhere - never listening or concentrating.

Zincum met. where there is marked agitation.

Acidity

A sensation of bitterness or acidity in the stomach, causing discomfort often associated with flatulence, heartburn and indigestion. It is often due to a faulty diet, emotional tension, and a faulty life-style.

REMEDIES

Carbo veg. for upper abdominal flatulence and discomfort.

Magnesium phos. for colicky pain.

Lycopodium the symptoms are mainly right-sided.

The above remedies should be taken three times daily until there is symptom relief.

Acne

The common chronic skin affection of teenagers and young adults. The exact cause is unknown but major contributing factors are stress, hormonal imbalance, poor and unbalanced diet, particularly one too rich in starchy and refined sugars. If not corrected the condition may lead to permanent scarring in later years.
REMEDIES
Graphites the acne oozes a clear fluid.
Kali brom. for an itchy acne with raised infected areas.
Sulphur for chronic problems, worse from heat or contact with water.
Where there is scarring, use such remedies as *Phytolacca, Thiosinaminum* or *Variolinum.*

Aconitum napellus (Monkshood)

One of the most acute remedies of all for colds and flu. It should be taken within the first 48 hours of onset. Especially indicated when symptoms are those of fear, pain, apprehension, restlessness and fear of dying. The symptoms often follow exposure to wind, rain or cold. The typical subject for *Aconitum* is of florid complexion and solid, well-built frame.

Acrocyanosis

A condition of peripheral cyanosis with a red or bluish tint to the peripheral extremities. Associated with poor circulation and coldness.
REMEDIES
Agaricus, Carbo veg., Lachesis.

Adhesions

These are a complication of either surgical intervention or previous infection. When healing occurs, fibrous scar tissue is laid down in the area affected causing distortion, sometimes blockage with interference to normal functioning.
REMEDIES
Bellis per., Graphites, Phytolacca, Staphysagria, Thiosinaminum.

Adolescent Depression

Depression of the teenage years, sometimes severe. There is often withdrawal from others into fantasy and a preoccupation with sexual problems, body imagery, hypochondriasis and guilt - often about masturbation.
REMEDIES
Lycopodium, Murex, Natrum mur.

Aerophagy

The common nervous habit in certain children and adults of constantly swallowing air when eating or on other occasions. This leads to symptoms of flatulence, fullness, indigestion and discomfort generally. Often the aerophagy is quite unconscious.
REMEDIES
Argentum nit., Carbo veg., Lycopodium.

Aesculus hippocastanum (Horse Chestnut)

Mainly a remedy for problems of the rectum and anal areas. Pain, congestion and discomfort are marked due to a combination of haemorrhoids and chronic constipation. Other common symptoms are:- anal prolapse, anal itching, sudden sharp and deep rectal pain or discomfort. It is of value for chronic symptoms in the area.

Aethusa (Fool's Parsley)

One of the major remedies for milk allergy in infants and children. Milk cannot be tolerated in any form, provoking vomiting soon after swallowing. The vomit is usually violent and projectile with curds which are 'shot out' as from a canon. In adults it is useful when there is an allergic condition to dairy products.

Agaricus amanita (Fly Agaric)

Indicated for confusional states including chronic alcoholism. Of special value in circulatory problems and helpful in chilblains or frost bite where there are red areas of burning, itching and swelling of fingers and toes. The extremities are cold, blue and painful.

Agoraphobia

Fear and panic at going out of doors alone or into any busy unfamiliar area. Usually there is a restricted feeling and fear of being held-up or delayed. All the symptoms are better for company and security. Having to wait in a queue, at a check-out point or traffic lights can often worsen anxiety. The cause is always profoundly psychological.
REMEDIES
Argentum nit., Lycopodium, Natrum mur., Pulsatilla.

Aggravation of Symptoms

This may occur in the course of homoeopathic treatment especially in the early stages. It often happens where the underlying problem has been suppressed over a period of time so that it is not readily available to the remedy's action. Homoeopathy appears to worsen the condition as it brings it to the surface. In this way it can be more easily and readily dealt with by the body as vital energy flows into the region making it more accessible to cure. Such aggravations are usually only transient aspects of early homoeopathic treatment and understood by the patient because they do not undermine the improved sense of well-being.

Ageing Problems

These are many and varied, but all centre around the general problem of degenerative changes. The commonest symptoms are loss of memory, confusion, anxiety, agitation, insomnia, arthritis and weakness. It is important to look at the whole picture of the individual concerned, including the quality of their diet, and any possible side-effects of prescribed drugs.
REMEDIES
Baryta carb., Carbo veg., Opium, Sulphur.

Agitation

The state of mental unrest, with fidgety restlessness and insomnia, often due to internal turmoil and anxiety.
REMEDIES
Argentum nit. panic and fear are the major causes.
Lycopodium fear of a future event provokes unrest.
Zinc met. the restlessness is mainly of the feet.

Agnus castus (Chaste Tree)

Although particularly effective in the sexual sphere, it is also a remedy for loss of vigour and drive where there is depression, disinterest and a weak response. For the male it is invaluable for impotence, weakness and inadequacy (compare *Silicea*). In the female it has a similar role where there is a diminished libidinal interest and activity, or sterility.

Air-Sickness

Symptoms of malaise, usually sickness, nausea, excessive salivation and dizziness occur when travelling by plane.

REMEDIES

Borax when the nausea occurs in an air-pocket with sudden downward movement.

Cocculus when dizziness and nausea are marked.

Pulsatilla when there is a psychological element strongly present, with apprehension made worse by noise or vibration.

Alcoholism

The common social addictive problem with excessive alcohol intake to compensate for feelings of underlying psychological inadequacy. There is often a strongly positive response to homoeopathy and remedies such as *Avena sat., Nux vom.,* may be required in high potency together with the constitutional prescription.

Aletris farinosa (Stargrass)

The remedy acts strongly upon the digestive system and reproductive organs. Indigestion, colicky pains and flatulence with nausea are common. The appetite is nil and the sight or thought of food stimulates nausea. Vomiting of pregnancy. The menstrual periods are heavy and excessive with clots and severe colicky pains. Also recommended for anaemia, exhaustion and recurrent miscarriages.

Allen, Henry C. M.D. (1836-1909)

The 19th century American homoeopathic physician and writer. He first (with Swan) described provings of *Lueticum* in *The Materia Medica of the Nosodes* with provings of *X-Ray* (Boericke and Tafel Phil. 1910). He taught at Chicago and was Dean of Hering College. President of the International Homoeopathic Association in 1886.
Major writings include:
Keynotes with Nosodes
Important Nosodes
Materia Medica of the Nosodes
The Therapeutics of Intermittent Fever

Allen, Timothy Field. M.D. (1837-1902)

The eminent 19th century American homoeopath, best known for his Encyclopedia of Pure Materia Medica in 10 volumes and still a standard quoted reference book. He worked mainly in Brooklyn, N.Y., where he was in practice. Born in Westminster, Vermont, he was the son of a doctor and also known as an organist and composer. In 1867 he became Professor of Anatomy at the New York Homoeopathic College and in 1871 Professor of Therapeutics and Materia Medica. He was Dean of the New York Homoeopathic Medical College. Allen worked as co-editor of the *New York Journal of Homoeopathy* and Director of the NY botanical garden. Major writings include:

1874 Encyclopedia of Pure Materia Medica
1876 Ophthalmic Therapeutics
1878 The Effects of Lead on Healthy Individuals
1880 A general symptom register of Homoeopathic Materia Medica
1889 A handbook of Materia Medica and Homoeopathic Therapeutics

Allergy

There is an acute antibody-reaction by the body to a protein element in the irritant which is treated as a foreign body and stimulates an inflammatory reaction. This may occur in asthma, hay-fever or following a bee or wasp sting.

REMEDIES

Rhus tox. reduces irritation, especially when a red rash is present.

Urtica urens given hourly in the acute attack is helpful to relieve swelling and irritation.

Allium cepa (Spanish onion)

The major symptoms are those of the common cold, with a streaming nasal watery discharge, itchy watering eyes, acute nasal catarrh, irritation and exhaustion. Useful in hay-fever and for coryza (common cold).

Allopathy

The system of conventional medicine, which differs from homoeopathy, by treating symptoms with their opposite in order to suppress them. When the patient is hot, he is given something to cool him down. When in pain - something to eradicate the pain and when agitated, a drug to calm him down. When over-calmed he is then given another drug to stimulate him. This is in direct contrast to the Homoeopathic approach which gives a 'like' remedy based on the Theory of Similars, to stimulate natural vital energy and a response in the area affected.

Aloe (the common aloe)

Mainly a rectal remedy for haemorrhoidal problems. There is restlessness and irritability. Chronic colicky diarrhoeal problems occur, with a tendency to soiling. Also for haemorrhoidal conditions which protrude and prolapse causing burning pain and congestion.

Alopecia

Loss of hair in circular or irregular patches in either sex. Male pattern baldness is hereditary in origin, but stress, drug side-effects and hormonal imbalance are other causes. More rarely the alopecia is total and may occur in children or adults - the cause unknown.
REMEDIES
Lycopodium, Vinca minor.

Alternative Medicine

Dr. Margery Blackie (see section) always said that Homeopathy was 'the' alternative medicine. It certainly offers a viable alternative to the conventional prescription for both patients and physician alike. But homoeopathy also acts in a complementary way to the conventional approach, and where a specific drug is essential, homoeopathy can still be used without interacting with the drug or inhibiting it. Much of conventional medicine is laboratory-based and largely synthetic, using products which suppress rather than conserve vital energy. Over-prescribing has become increasingly common and is responsible for much of the present dissatisfaction with the health service approach to community health.

Alumina (the metal Aluminium - as its oxide)

The main indications are chronic and absolute constipation, often where manual removal of faeces is required. Also for eczema and 'itchy eyes'. Because they may be a trigger to constipation or allergy, the use of aluminium utensils in the kitchen should be avoided.

Ammonium muriaticum (Sal Ammoniac)

A remedy for paralysing exhausting symptoms, nearly always worse first thing in the mornings. The make-up is sluggish, oedematous and obese, with slowness in all areas of the digestive system. Depression may occur, also headache at the root of the nose. The head feels bruised. Scalp irritation and chronic problems of scalp-eczema and dandruff are other indications.

Ammonium phosphoricum (Phosphate of Ammonia)

The titration of the organic salt, first proved by Voigt. A remedy for chronic problems, particularly recurrent gout, poor circulation and facial paralysis. It acts on the hands and feet where there are chronic gouty arthritic problems with swelling, nodular formation and pain.

Amnesia

Loss of memory associated with fatigue and poor concentration *(Lycopodium). A* head injury, however remote, that first caused the problem suggests *Helleborus.* When there is shock of any kind, give Arnica. Hysterical amnesia responds well to *Gelsemium* or *Ignatia.* When due to senility, ***Baryta carb*** may improve the condition.

Amyl nitrosum (Amyl Nitrate)

A major remedy for flashes of heat and tension in the head with anxiety, sweating and palpitations. Such symptoms occur at the menopause and afterwards causing distress. They can also occur in a younger person - either male or female, with over-sensitivity, painful sweating, a sensation of heat and head fullness. The patient has tachycardia, pulse irregularity and chest pain of the anginal type radiating down the arm or up into the neck area. Flushing, throbbing and violent heart-beating are other symptoms (compare *Belladonna).*

Anacardium orientale (Marking nut)

A remedy for chronic digestive problems associated with pain and fullness after meals, but relieved by further eating. Constipation is severe and chronic. There are many odd, bizarre and hypochondriacal facets to the remedy in particular the symptom of the inside or uterus feeling 'blocked by a plug', or there is a girdle or hoop encircling the body. Weakness is associated. The bizarre ideas may be psychotic and delusional.

Anaemia

There is usually deficiency of the iron-containing blood element haemoglobin which binds and transports oxygen to the cells. When this is lacking, symptoms of exhaustion, pallor and shortness of breath occur. The cause may be haemorrhage, from a variety of causes, particularly piles or a heavy menstrual loss. It can occur in pregnancy and also from dietary insufficiency. Other kinds of anaemia also occur, such as Pernicious anaemia (vitamin B12 deficiency), Sickle cell and Folic acid anaemia. The homoeopath will always base his approach on the symptoms of the individual patient and the whole person, rather than solely relying on the pathology or the cause. But he will also take this into account and he may give Folic acid in homoeopathic potency when he feels this is indicated for the individual as a totality.

REMEDIES

Ferrum met. is indicated for an iron-deficiency anaemia, but the underlying cause must always be carefully diagnosed and treated.

Angina Pectoris

There is a heavy constricting pain across the chest and sometimes up into the neck or down the arms. The cause is usually due to insufficient blood supply to the heart due to arteriosclerosis of the coronary arteries supplying the heart muscle. Pain is typically worse for physical effort or stress, but relieved by rest.
REMEDIES
Arsenicum alb., Cactus, Latrodectus, Nux vomica.

Animal Experiments

These are not used in the testing or 'proving' of homoeopathic remedies - traditionally carried out on healthy human volunteers. In recent years a few European animal research experiments have been carried out to demonstrate the efficiency of certain remedies in potency on the regeneration of liver-cells poisoned by a toxic substance. However, these are the exception and homoeopathy is mainly based on symptoms recorded by the healthy human. Clinical observation studies and toxicology are the other factors which form the repertory or reference of symptoms.

Anorexia Nervosa

The common emotional illness of adolescent girls where there is a preoccupation with weight loss, body image and compulsive food intake. Dieting may be so severe, that health and life are threatened. The underlying psychological attitudes in both patient and family must be explored.
REMEDIES
Natrum mur., Pulsatilla, Sulphur.

Anthracinum (Anthrax)

Prepared from the anthrax-infected spleen of sheep, and first introduced by Lux (see section). It is an important and valuable remedy, particularly where there is a severe infection, boil or carbuncle with pus and burning pains.

Antidotes to Homoeopathic Remedies

On rare occasions a patient is unable to tolerate the homoeopathic vital reaction because it is too strong, or the remedy may bring to the surface an earlier problem that is felt to be overwhelming. In such cases the remedy can be neutralised or antidoted by its specific antidote. In most cases *Camphora* or *Sulphur* can be used to neutralise a remedy given unwisely after an improvement and leading to a reaction, often a proving symptom in a sensitive person, instead of leaving the single dose to complete the cure. The persistent use of coffee or tea during homoeopathic treatment lessens its effect and may neutralise the action of the remedies. If remedies are stored close to camphor, or strong perfume, this will also render them ineffective. Taking a course of steroid remedies at the same time as a homoeopathic remedy, will tend to either neutralise the homoeopathic response, or severely restrict it.

Antimonium tartaricum (Tartar Emetic)

An acute remedy for inflammatory conditions, particularly effective in chest conditions where there is an accumulation of fluid and a loud rattling cough with laboured breathing, as in asthma or bronchitis.

Anxiety States

The increasingly common psychological state of fear and insecurity, not usually linked to an external event yet sufficient to provoke a severe response.
REMEDIES
Argentum nitricum when associated with fear.
Ignatia when linked with grief.
Lycopodium for marked hypochondriacal tendencies.
Natrum mur where there is marked tension.
Pulsatilla useful for marked tearfulness.
Nux vomica or *Sepia* for associated snappy irritability.

Aphasia (post stroke)

Loss of speech following a stroke. *Arnica* 30 three times daily is recommended until improvement occurs.

Apis mellifica (The Honey Bee)

The source is the whole crushed bee. The action is rapid and dramatic particularly indicated for acute condition with swelling, restlessness, redness, stinging pain, itching, and acute discomfort. A characteristic of the remedy is the marked absence of any desire to pass water and the lack of thirst. (Compare with *Pulsatilla* which has the same absence of thirst).

Apomorphia (The morphine alkaloid derivative)

A remedy to be considered for states of severe and chronic vomiting sometimes occurring without nausea. Sweating, fainting and weakness with giddiness is characteristic. Of value in alcoholism, drug abuse, also for vomiting of pregnancy.

Appetite Excess

There is an excessive and constant craving to eat or to pick at food at any opportunity, the appetite never appeased. The underlying reason is often one of stress and tension, the patient turning to food particularly sweet foods for comfort and relief. In chronic miasmic disease of the Psora type it is a particular feature, when *Sulphur* may be indicated. In others, the craving is for sweet things like chocolate where *Lycopodium* is the best remedy. Salt taken excessively, indicates *Natrum mur* as a possible remedy. Once the underlying causative factors are clear then *Phytolacca berry* is useful to control the appetite craving.

Appetite Loss

The loss of desire or interest in food. This may be a symptom of many acute conditions - often an infection during the incubation stage of measles or chicken-pox or where there is a raised temperature. It is also common in many chronic debilitating illnesses as hepatitis or glandular fever. After a severe cold or flu', *Nux vomica* 6 is particularly useful. For stress-related conditions, conditions of energy or appetite loss, *Kali phos.*6 is helpful.

Argentum nitricum (Silver Nitrate)

Nitrate of silver in a triturated solution. Its main indications are panic and anxiety states, particularly of the agoraphobic type. There is fear of failure and criticism by others as with a public speaking engagement, examinations, interviews, also stage fright. The remedy always has the most absolute intolerance of heat of any remedy (compare *Pulsatilla*). Abdominal flatulence and distension are commonly present (compare *Carbo veg., Lycopodium).*

Arnica (Leopard's Bane)

Arnica takes its source from the Fall-Kraut plant grown in the Alps at altitudes over 5,000 feet. It is one of the most useful and fundamental of all homoeopathic remedies and should be present in every family medical chest. Its action is specific for bruising and shock and it is the major remedy for sprains with pain, inflammation and swelling. Shock from any cause, as after childbirth or dental extraction, responds well reducing recovery time and side-effects. When there has been a trauma of any kind - forceps at childbirth, accident or injury, before and after surgery, *Arnica* makes the passage more comfortable and the recovery period shorter.

Arsenicum album (White trioxide of Arsenic)

Source is white arsenic oxide in homoeopathic potency. One of the polycrest remedies of multiple action, it is an acute remedy acting particularly on the chest and alimentary tract where there is restlessness, burning pains, craving for heat, chilliness, breathlessness or diarrhoea. Like *Arnica* it is one of the most useful of the homoeopathic remedies and should be in every family medical box in the home and taken on holidays, for emergency use.

Arteriosclerosis

Hardening of the arteries of the elderly, but increasingly present in younger age groups (as discovered at autopsies of U.S. Marine combat troops of the Korean war). The incidence was surprisingly high - up to 30% in many young soldiers. It is associated with diets high in animal fat and cholesterol, prolonged breast feeding of the male infant (a year or longer), high levels of cigarette smoking and stress, but the exact cause is still unknown.

REMEDIES

Agaricus, Baryta carb., Cactus, Carbo veg., the individual Constitutional remedy.

Arthritis

This may be osteo-arthritic or rheumatoid type. The former is due basically to wear and tear and may involve any joint, but it is particularly the large joints of knee, hip or spine which are most affected. Rheumatoid arthritis is a more generalised inflammatory condition involving small and large joints, especially the elbow, wrist and hand.

REMEDIES

Apis is indicated for painful swelling.

Belladonna for redness, heat and swelling with pain.

Bryonia is called for when symptoms are aggravated by heat and movement.

Causticum is indicated for certain types of neck arthritis and when there is paralysis and wasting.

Medorrhinum for more chronic intractable conditions.

Rhus tox. where there is stiffness, better for movement and heat, worse for damp.

Sanguinaria for arthritis of the shoulder joint.

Arum triphyllum (Jack-in-the-Pulpit)

Its main action is on the mucous membrane of the nasal passages. There is blockage due to catarrh, with a bitter irritating pungent discharge and causing a bright red raw soreness of the nostril area. Mouth breathing is characteristic. The mouth, lips and throat are raw and uncomfortable, the voice unpredictable, due to an associated laryngitis. It is often helpful for singers, orators or actors, where there is damage to the vocal chords from excessive use and strain. The hoarseness is worse from singing. There is a tendency to constantly pick at the nasal and lip areas and cause bleeding. All symptoms are aggravated by cold and exposure to winds, also from lying down. It is often indicated for a very severe viral common cold (coryza) and in scarlet fever.

Asafoetida (Stinkasand)

A remedy for chronic hysterical problems often with a depressive origin to them, chronic indigestion with aerophagy, flatulence and distension, an impression of having a lump in the throat (Compare *Natrum mur).* Variability of all symptoms and of mental attitudes generally (compare *Pulsatilla).*

Astacus fluviatilis (Crawfish)

A remedy for allergy, particularly when there is a severe urticarial skin reaction after eating shellfish. The rash is red and may involve the whole body, with intolerable itching and swelling of the lymph glands. It is common to have a raised temperature, feeling chilly and sensitive to the least draught of cold air.

Asthma

The common condition of acute bronchospasm which is common in childhood or in the early 40's as late-onset asthma. The condition may be acute or chronic with marked shortness of breath, wheezing, apprehension and restlessness. Asthma often has a familial tendency to involve the shy sensitive personality with allergic tendencies. Many cases are now thought to be linked to atmospheric traffic pollution.
REMEDIES
Arsenicum, Bryonia, Kali carb., Medorrhinum, Phosphorus, Tub bov.

Atropinum (Atropine)

Atropine is an alkaloid derivative of *Belladonna.* It acts on the nervous system, causing delirium, the pupils dilated, redness of the face and upper half of the body, vomiting of milk, double vision and distortion of objects, which seem too large or elongated. Other symptoms which indicate the remedy are:- dryness of the throat, swallowing difficulties and burning irritation in the pit of the stomach. Stiffness of the left leg and left knee and the right great toe.

Aurum Metallicum (the metal Gold)

A remedy which is especially indicated for chronic or recurrent depressive problems with suicidal despair. There are many cardiac problems associated, with palpitations, angina pectoris, often severe painful arthritic conditions with hip and knee disability. It is a remedy of immense importance and value.

Avena sativa (the Oat)

Made from a tincture of the fresh flowering whole plant. Indications are extreme nervous prostration, impotence, palpitations, lack of concentration and insomnia. It is a useful remedy in drug addiction and alcoholism.

B

Baby-problems

These respond well to the correct homoeopathic prescription. A clear diagnosis must be made in every case of the cause of each symptom.
REMEDIES
Aethusa for projectile vomiting.
Borax cries when put down.
Carbo veg. mainly flatulence with abdominal distension (Also consider *Lycopodium).*
Chamomilla cries from anger when teething. Not thriving or failing to gain weight needs careful consideration and diagnosis.
Silicea excessive wind.

Bach, Edward. M.D., D.P.H. (1886 - 1936)

Originally a pathologist and bacteriologist, Bach always took an active interest in the problems of treating chronic disease. He began working on the bowel nosodes from vaccines of intestinal bacteria, giving them orally, in homoeopathic potencies with positive results, especially for chronic problems e.g. arthritis. He became convinced of the healing properties of nature and the therapeutic value of various tinctures of wild flowers, especially Impatiens, Mimulus and Clematis, which are still widely used in Rescue Remedy. Although not a homoeopath, he was a gifted healer and inspired researcher who developed an alternative philosophy and a system of healing.
Major writings include:
Heal Thyself
Free Thyself

Twelve Healers
Chronic Disease (Co-author, Dr. C.W. Wheeler)

Backward Child

The child is retarded in development and not attaining the normal expected milestones - both physically and mentally for his age. The causes are often obscure. These include birth trauma, genetic abnormalities, infection during the early developmental months of pregnancy, constitutional or familial factors, mainly miasmic in type, especially psora. There may be a physical congenital deformity of the heart or vascular system. Down's Syndrome (mongolism) is another common factor.
REMEDIES
Baryta carb. more indicated for the dull, heavily built child, obviously slow and backward, looking more 'mental' and a tendency to enlarged glands and sore throats.
Capsicum for the backward child who is always homesick.
Medorrhinum for Down's syndrome (mongolism).
Natrum mur. for the difficult backward child with behaviour problems, late in walking and with a tendency to sleep-walking.
Staphysagria where the child is extremely resentful but vulnerable and easily hurt and sensitive.
Tuberculinum bov. for children who are spiteful and resentful, but always better for travelling.

Backache

Lumbago is low backache due to a combination of cold or damp together with muscle spasm. It is very painful and incapacitating. Sacro-iliac pain is often due to ligamental strain with local tenderness, aching pain and sometimes sciatica. A prolapsed inter-vertebral disc causes severe, sometimes paralysing pain, which is usually incapacitating. Vertebral displacement is a mechanical problem that initially needs osteopathic correction. It often causes shortening of one leg and 'tilting' of the pelvis. If shortening is permanent, one shoe may need building-up and adjusting.
REMEDIES
Bryonia, Causticum, Medorrhinum, Natrum mur., Nux vomica, Radium brom., Rhus tox., Ruta, Sulphur.

Bacillus No V11 (Paterson)

The bowel nosode, and 7th non-lactose fermenting organism which Paterson discovered in the laboratory. Its main indications are mental and physical exhaustion, as occurs in post-viral syndromes (M.E.). Flatulence and a sense of fullness occurs after eating. Libido is weak, with a poor or weak urinary flow. Other symptoms which indicate the remedy are:- a weak chest with a tendency to asthma or bronchitis, rheumatic fibrositis - causing pains in the back, neck, shoulders or arms. The pulse is slow, blood-pressure low. Premature senility is another indication for this nosode. It is closely related to *Kali carb.*

Balance (Internal)

This is an essential aspect of health especially at a psychological level. It is often only after the internal harmony has been upset by stress, shock, or poor nutrition, diminishing resistance and the vital force, that illness occurs. The tissues quickly become vulnerable to invasion and illness as their intrinsic vitality is lessened. Symptoms often only appear at a much later stage, although malaise, fatigue, exhaustion and irritability are common early manifestations of imbalance.

Barriers to Cure

These are relevant when the homoeopathic remedy fails to effect the expected vital response. There may be antidoting of the remedies by the use of an allopathic suppressant treatment at the same time as the homoeopathic one, especially steroids or antibiotics. The excessive use of coffee, tea or cigarettes can reduce the efficiency of homoeopathic treatment. The remedy may have been neutralised and made ineffective by storage in excessive sunlight or heat, near camphor or strong perfumes. Excessive handling of the remedies also undermines their efficiency. An underlying miasm may be present, especially in chronic disease and makes the expected treatment less efficient. Sometimes the patient, if repeatedly taking homoeopathic remedies, based on unwise self-prescribing, prevents the prescribed remedy from being effective. A final factor and an important one is that there is a mechanical barrier to cure, which requires either manipulation or surgery to relieve it.

Bed wetting (Enuresis)

There is a lack of control over bladder-functioning by the growing child at the expected time, so that bed-wetting continues uncontrollably, often into the teens. It is far more common in boys than girls. The condition may have existed since infancy, bladder control never attained at night, or in some conditions it was established early and then lost following a psychological shock or threat to security - as with a new baby. There may also be a familiar (genetic) factor, one parent also late in establishing bladder control.
REMEDIES
Calcarea carb., Equisetum, Lycopodium, Pulsatilla.

Belladonna (Deadly Nightshade)

The acute remedy for inflammatory conditions marked by heat, redness, pain, tenderness sensitivity and restlessness. The condition may affect the ears with acute otitis media, the throat with acute tonsillitis or the skin with scarlet fever. The sensitivity is such that the very least jarring movement or draught of cold air provokes irritation and an aggravation of the condition.

Bellis perennis (Daisy)

A remedy for severe chronic sprains with damage to muscular fibres and tendons. Useful after *Arnica* when the condition persists and there is pain or discomfort and stiffness. For strain and tendon injury due to excessive effort, when caught off balance, or pain from a false movement, sudden cold or chill. Fatigue, chill and swelling are marked and diagnostic.

Benjamin, Alva. M.D. (1884-1975)

The distinguished homoeopathic practitioner, formerly secretary-general of the International League and later president. Treasurer of the Faculty Council at the Royal London Homoeopathic Hospital for many years. A graduate of Sydney University, he was physician at the Royal London Homoeopathic Hospital from 1923-56 with a special interest in dermatology. In 1958 he founded the Hahnemann Society.

Benzoic acidum (Benzoic acid)

Indicated for arthritic and urinary complaints. The urine is scanty, dark brown (with no deposit) and a strong offensive odour. It is helpful for dribbling of the elderly, cystitis and changeable gouty rheumatic problems, especially of the knees, wrist and the achilles tendon. Also for uterine prolapse, menstrual problems and asthma.

Berberis vulgaris (Barberry)

A major renal remedy. Pain and frequency are the major indications. Renal colic is commonly relieved. There is often distortion of perspective so that other people appear to be larger, or the head itself feels bigger, enclosed in a tight-fitting cap. The remedy may also be helpful for renal (kidney) stones.

Berridge, Edward W. M.D. (1878 - 1921)

The English physician and graduate of Pennsylvania Homoeopathic college, founder of the International Homoeopathic Association and formerly resident medical officer to the Liverpool Homoeopathic Dispensary. He is important because he was one of the earliest homoeopaths, treating Dr. Thomas Skinner (see section) with high-potency remedies and instrumental in convincing him of the therapeutic merits of homoeopathy. Later he became his tutor. He was a co-editor of *The Organon journal* with Lippe, Skinner and Swan.

Major writings include:

1869 *Complete Repertory of the Homoeopathic Materia Medica Diseases of the Eye*

Bites

If extensive and lacerating, clean locally with *Calendula*, give *Arnica* 30, followed by *Staphisagria* 6 hourly. Hospitalise the patient. When small and penetrating, give *Hypericum* and *Ledum*. Snake bites may require hospitalisation. When the bite is from a dog that is suspected of rabies, give homoeopathic *Lyssin* 30 daily until symptoms have subsided.

Blackie, Margery Grace. M.D.,C.V.0., F.F.Hom. (1898-1981)

Probably the most well-known and respected homoeopath of recent years who has done so much to make Homoeopathy more widely appreciated in the past decades. Graduate of the Royal Free Hospital, Dean of the Faculty of Homoeopathy, great-niece of Dr. Compton-Burnett, she was physician to the Royal household from 1969. Her 50 years of practise were at all times an example for both patients and students alike. She was a close colleague of Dr.Frank Bodman (see section) and they had remained close friends since the 20's when both served under Dr. D. Borland as house-physicians. She was an able lecturer, supporter of research, country lover and enjoyed relaxing with a jig-saw-puzzle. A 'high' prescriber in Kentian (see section) traditions, she also taught the single, unrepeated-remedy traditional and pure approach to homoeopathy to the benefit of her many patients. Her Kensington fork-supper parties during the Faculty meetings are still be fresh in the memory of many. In her general style and approach to homoeopathy, she was a joy to observe. She inaugurated the Blackie Research Trust and this continues her traditions. Many of her lectures are recorded on tape.

Major writing include:

1977 The Patient, not the Cure

1986 Classical Homoeopathy

Bladder Problems

Infections (Pain, irritation) - see Cystitis

Blockage - see Retention of urine

Haemorrhage - see Haematuria

Stones - see Calculus

Bleeding (Haemorrhage)

Loss of blood from any part of the body - either of spontaneous or traumatic causation - other than normal menstrual loss. In all cases the flow must be stopped and any shock to the general condition must have priority. With bleeding from a wound or cut, arrest the flow by pressure locally. Give *Arnica* for shock, and use *Calendula* locally.

REMEDIES

Arnica for nose bleeding (epistaxis) - every few minutes until bleeding stops.

Aconitum when due to heat or raised blood-pressure, in a thick-set individual.

Pulsatilla when there is a recurrent tendency to nose-bleeds, the temperament passive, worse for heat, occurring in the latter part of the day.

Ferrum phos. is a very useful remedy for haemorrhage, where there is prostration and anaemia, the remedy increasing the haemoglobin levels.

Hamamelis is indicated for bleeding from haemorrhoids. Also consider *Aesculus.*

Blisters

Commonly due to friction from ill-fitting shoe or excessive local pressure or rubbing and causing damage to the skin.

REMEDIES

Apis when there is less fluid with considerable soreness of surrounding tissues, also following a bee or wasp sting.

Cantharis where there is a persistence of burning discomfort, redness and pain.

Mercurius when the blisters are infected.

Urtica is useful when there is much swelling with irritation, or when allergic in origin.

Use the nosode if the blisters are part of a chicken-pox rash.

Bodman, Francis Hervey. M.D. (1900 - 1980)

The homoeopathic physician who studied with Dr. Blackie under Borland and Wheeler (see section), working initially as a houseman to the Royal London Homoeopathic Hospital and later in Bristol where he established his practice. He had a D.P.M. (Diploma of Psychological Medicine) as well as the homoeopathic degree. His stimulating, frequently erudite writings and communications always contained a sensitive awareness of the importance of the mental and psychological aspects of the patient.

Boenninghausen, Clemens M.F. von. M.D. (1785-1864)

Born in Heringhaven, Holland, he first qualified as a lawyer following family traditions and was only introduced to homoeopathy by chance. A serious fall led to a purulent tuberculous local condition of such a degree that in 1828, his life and health was in danger. He was however cured by a friend and later colleague, Dr. Weihe who used homoeopathy and converted him to the importance and significance of the method. From that time he became a most active supporter and promoter of homoeopathy through lectures and writings. His fame became such, that in 1843 he was given a license by Royal decree to practise homoeopathy, although not as a physician. In 1854 he received an honourary M.D. from the Cleveland Homoeopathic College. He corresponded regularly with Hahnemann throughout his life and they were close friends. Dr. Carol Dunham, the eminent homoeopath of that time was also a close friend and supporter.
Major writings include:
1845 Essay on the homoeopathic treatment of Intermittent Fever
1847 Boenninghausen's therapeutic pocket-book for homoeopathics

1847 The sides of the body and drug affinities
1860 The homoeopathic treatment of whooping cough
1833 Homoeopathic therapy of intermittent fevers
Characteristics of homoeopathic remedies

Boericke, Francis Edmund. M.D. (1826 - 1901)

Born in Glauchus Germany, Boericke settled in America, obtaining in 1863 his M.D. from the Homoeopathic Medical College of Pennsylvania. He was lecturer at the Hahnemann Medical College in Pharmacy. He is primarily known for establishing with his brother-in-law Adolph Tafel, the Boericke and Tafel homoeopathic pharmacy in the US. In addition he formed the well known and highly regarded Boericke Publishing Company.

Boericke, William. M.D. (1849-1929)

The eminent American homoeopathic physician. Born in Czechoslovakia and nephew of F.E. Boericke. Graduate of the Philadelphia Medical College in 1880, he studied for a year in Vienna before moving to San Francisco where he worked as a homoeopath for 50 years. He was founder of the *California Homoeopath* journal, which later became the *Pacific Coast Journal of Homoeopathy* and a founder of the Hahnemann Medical College of the Pacific in San Francisco 1881. President of the California State Homoeopathic Society. Major writings include:
Stepping Stones to Homoeopathic Health
1888 The Twelve Tissue Remedies
1912 Principles of Homoeopathy
Management and Care of Children
His Homoeopathic Materia Medica and Repertory

reached nine editions (1927) and is still an everyday standard reference for many. He also translated the important sixth edition of the *Organon* from the complicated German text.

Boger, Cyrus M. M.D. (1861-1935)

The 19th century homoeopathic practitioner, graduate of the Philadelphia Hahnemann College in 1888. President of the International Homoeopathic Association 1904. Major writings include:
Synoptic Key to Materia Medica
Additions to Kent's Repertory
Boenninghausen's Characteristics
A Systematic Alphabetic repertory of homoeopathic remedies
Times of the remedies and the moon phases

Bone Pains

This may be an aspect of injury or arthritis. The recommended remedy is *Symphytum* 6c three times daily.

Borax (Borate of Sodium)

The remedy has its major action on the intestinal tract and is helpful for nausea, vomiting, abdominal pains, and diarrhoea. Dizziness and sweating is marked. All symptoms are typically aggravated by downward motion in any form.

Borland, Douglas. M.D. (1885-1960)

The eminent teacher and prescriber who influenced so many contemporary homoeopathic practitioners. Born in Glasgow and a graduate from there, he was an outstanding teacher, prescriber and lecturer. He was on the staff of the Royal London Homoeopathic Hospital. He came to America in 1908 with Weir and Fergie-Woods (see section) studying under Kent, on a Tyler scholarship. From 1945 he became governor of the London Homoeopathic Hospital. He was also president of the Homoeopathic Society. His monogram on children's types is still widely read and referred to and has become a classic. He was an advocate of high potency prescribing in England and the important Kentian (see section) tradition of the single dose.
Posthumous writings include:-
Homoeopathy in Practice.

Bovista (Warted Puff-Ball)

The remedy for disordered speech including stammering and stuttering. It helps many chronic skin problems with oozing eczema, urticaria, corns and warts. The chronic eruptions have a crust and itch severely. All symptoms are worse for heat. (Compare *Pulsatilla, Argentum nit., Sulphur).*

Bowel Nosodes

Developed initially by the bacteriologist Dr. Edward Bach and later by Drs. John and Elizabeth Paterson who researched a series of nosodes from the non-lactose fermenting *B.Coli* bowel organisms. They are enormously important in treatment, especially of chronic disease. The major bowel nosodes are :- *Morgan, Proteus, Caertner, Dys. Co., Sycotic Co.*

Boyd, William Ernest. M.D. (1891-1955)

Dr. Boyd studied medicine, lived and practised in Glasgow throughout his life. He was an eminent practitioner and thinker who combined the sensitivity of a physician with the practical approach of a research engineer. As a young man he was particularly impressed by the work of Dr. Robert Gibson-Miller and eventually became committed to the homoeopathic method. He was physician to the Glasgow Homoeopathic hospital from 1920. Using concepts of electro-physics, he invented the emanometer to demonstrate the measurable force in homoeopathic potencies and to match this with 'emanations' from patient's tissues-fluids to select remedies.
He also carried out physiological and biochemical research and published many papers in the British Homoeopathic Journal.
Major writings include:
1954 Biochemical and Biological Evidence of the Activity of High Potencies (B.H.J.).

Breasts - painful

When the problem is located in the nipple with acute inflammation, take *Aconite* 6 hourly until relief occurs. Use *Hepar sulph.* if sore and cracked. *Merc. sol.* is effective when there is burning pain and marked swelling with a deep-seated infection.

Pain may occur because of an abscess in the breast tissue, usually during lactation.

REMEDIES
Aconitum for very acute cases,
Bryonia when the breast is hard and painful.
Hepar sulph. when there is obvious pus formation with throbbing pains and a raised temperature.
Sulphur when the problem is at a more skin level, with rubbing, chaffing, and chapped skin.

Breathing difficulties

Usually these take the form of either shortness of breath or wheezing. In all cases the underlying reason must be very carefully diagnosed and any mechanical or obstructive cause dealt with. Chronic bronchitis and emphysema is one of the commonest causes and responds to remedies which stimulate the vital energies of the lungs. These include *Natrum sulph., Bryonia, Phosphorus, Arsenicum, Antimonium tart.* Wheezing may be due to several factors including asthma, bronchitis or a foreign body. The causes must be carefully explored and any allergic factors dealt with. Anxiety must also be taken into account as a possible trigger to attacks.
REMEDIES
House dust, Kali carb., Medorrhinum, Phosphorus.

Brittle nails

The nails are hard, without strength and are fragile tending to split and crack very easily - either downwards or across.
REMEDIES
Natrum mur. for hard, brittle nails which break or crack
Silicea especially where there is a tendency towards 'hang-nail' infection of the finger tips.

Bronchitis

There is an infection, either acute, or recurrent and chronic, of the lining mucosal layer of the bronchial tubes. When chronic there may be mucosal thickening with yellow or white phlegm coughed up. Asthma with bronchospasm is commonly associated.
REMEDIES
Bryonia, Hepar sulph., Medorrhinum, Sulphur, Tub.bov.

Bronchopneumonia

Acute inflammation of lung tissue, usually of the lung bases and often viral in origin, although sometimes bacterial in type. The onset can be very acute, often in an apparently fit strong person. There is a high temperature, shortness of breath and collapse. When the condition involves the elderly the temperature may be normal, because of a reduced vital reaction and antibiotics may also be needed.
REMEDIES
Antimonium tart., Arsenicum, Lycopodium, Mercurius, Pyrogen.

Bryonia (Wild Hops)

The important remedy which has its major action on the alimentary tract and mucous membrane. It is especially helpful for acute conditions with dryness and discomfort on movement. It also acts deeply on the joints. Pains are typically stitch-like, and often aggravated by both heat and movement but better for rest. The patient immobilises the affected area by lying on it as the least movement causes pain and irritation.

Bunions

There is chronic low-grade inflammation of the first or proximal metatarso-phalangeal joint of the great toe associated with swelling, pain, redness and painful thickening of the area. In most cases it is caused by either wear-and-tear of the joint (e.g. a sport's injury), or tight, ill-designed and poor fitting shoes. Obesity and a poor posture are other causative factors.
REMEDIES.
Hekla Lava is also useful to lessen the swelling once the acute inflammatory process has quietened down.
Rhus tox. when the condition is part of a general arthritic or rheumatic process.
Silicea the feet are cold, and sweating is profuse.

Burnett, James Compton. M.D. (1840-1901)

One of the most famous and prolific writers of all the English homoeopaths of the last century. Great-uncle of Dr. Margery Blackie, his ability to communicate and explain the working principles and clinical results of homoeopathy did much to stimulate serious interest in the profession. He was an 'organ' (the emphasis on disease in a specific area) prescriber and supporter of Rademacher's (see section) teachings.
Major writings include:
1881 The prevention of Congenital Malformation defects
1894 *Gout and its Cure*
1894 On fistula
1882 Cataract - causes and curability
1892 Fifty Reasons for being a Homoeopath
1882 Curability of Cataract
1890 Diseases of the Liver
1898 Change of Life in Women

Burns

When severe give *Arnica* 30 every hour for shock and hospitalise the patient immediately in a specialised burns unit. When only mild and localised, without shock, give *Arnica* 6 three times daily, or *Cantharis* 6 for severe pain. *Hypericum* or *Calendula* cream can be applied locally. In more severe cases the area is best kept dry and exposed to clean air, the patient in bed and quiet. For blistering give *Urtica urens* 6c for redness and swelling or *Belladonna* 6c followed by *Sulphur* 6c if the patient is not quickly made more comfortable in 24 hours. When extensive, or if in any doubt at all hospitalise immediately.

C

Cactus grandiflorus (Night-blooming Cereus)

The important remedy for tight constricting pain - particularly of the heart in anginal conditions. The typical pain is like a tight band and often there are palpitations and anxiety with a sense of oppression. Haemorrhages also occur, both nasal and anal.

Caladium seguinum (American Arum)

Indicated for genital itching (pruritis). The genital area is swollen and irritated. Sweating is marked. It is a remedy for impotency, also useful for asthma associated with excessive smoking. All symptoms are worse from movement, better for rest and sleep.

Calcarea carbonica (Calcium Carbonate)

One of the most important of all the polycrest remedies. Indicated for chronic disease of the psora type with chill, sweating, lack of vital response, weakness and obsessional mannerisms.

Calcarea fluorica (Fluoride of Lime)

Indicated for localised stony hard areas, particularly of the breast, but also in the lymph nodes. Also for gouty arthritic areas of the fingers, wrists, tendons or ligaments. Indicated for varicose veins, rickets, arteriosclerosis, cataract and to prevent post-operative adhesions.

Calcarea hypophosphorosa (Hypophospite of Lime)

Of special value in the *Calcarea* type of make-up with typical chill, pallor and coldness, with chronic arthritic conditions or rheumatism of the hands which are damp, weak or cold, worse for humid, chilly conditions.

Calcarea iodata (lodide of Lime)

For chronic glandular infections of the cervical region, especially tonsillar problems or goitre. Also for adenoidal problems and fibrous tumours of the breast or uterus.

Calcarea phosphorica (Phosphate of Lime)

Indicated for chronic weakness and pallor in a slim person of delicate constitution, with marked weakness especially in the mental areas and where bone development has been interfered with by trauma or surgery. Burning pains of the *Phosphorus* type with weakness and sweating give the diagnostic clue.

Calcarea sulphurica (Plaster of Paris, Gypsum)

For chronic infected skin conditions in the *Calcarea* type of make-up with weakness, obesity and thick catarrh. Infection discharging pus, the skin looks dirty often grey and usually feels damp and chilly.

Calculus (Stones)

These may occur in the gall-bladder or bile duct. They may cause severe colicky pain with vomiting and collapse, sometimes associated with jaundice. Attention should be paid to the diet, avoiding fatty foods high in saturated fats and those rich in oxalate, especially strawberries and spinach.

REMEDIES

Aconitum, Berberis, Chelidonium, China (helps prevent a re-occurrence), *Mercurius, Nux vomica.*

Stones also occur in the kidney, ureter or bladder, where they can cause very severe colicky pain with nausea, vomiting and collapse. Renal colic can be recurrent as small gravel stones are passed along the ureter to the bladder.

REMEDIES

Belladonna, Berberis, Nux vomica, Oxalic ac., Pareira, Phosphoric ac., Sarsaparilla.

Calendula officinalis (Marigold)

A remedy for wounds, cuts, infection, boils or carbuncle. It may be used locally as an ointment or tincture, or taken in potency - usually in the 6c potency. It acts to stimulate and provoke healing and lessens pus formation and infection, helping drainage of any infected area. It is basic to all first-aid treatment.

Camphora (Camphor)

A remedy for acute states of collapse with shock, pallor, chill and marked sweating, yet intolerance of any form of covering, such as a coat or blanket. Anxiety is marked with spasm and sometimes convulsions. Nausea, great coldness, low blood-pressure, though less sweating than *Veratrum alb.*, which closely resembles it. This remedy is useful if *Arnica* has failed to elicit a response.

Cannabis indica (Hashish)

A remedy for disturbed states of mind with dreamy unreality, hallucinations, disturbances of sensation and perspective. It is useful in psychotic conditions and for the ill effects of drug abuse - never well since that time, particularly after excessive marijuana. It is no longer prescribable in the U.K.

Cannabis sativa (Hemp)

Mainly a remedy for ocular problems with lens opacity as cataract. There are also powerful irritating urinary symptoms with burning pains, urgency and spasm as occurs in severe cystitis or urethritis (compare *Sycotic Co.*). It is no longer prescribable in the U.K.

Cantharis (Spanish Fly)

The remedy for acute irritating conditions of the mucous membrane, especially of the bladder where burning raw pains of excruciating intensity give the indication to prescribe. Indicated when a severe cystitis gives no rest. It is active in conditions of acute burning pain and this includes the skin, as after a scald, burn or severe infective condition (compare *Belladonna*).

Carbo animalis (Animal Charcoal)

A remedy for the elderly, resembling *Baryta carb.* because of its ability to stimulate a vital reaction in broken-down chronic conditions with poor circulation and exhaustion. Chronic bronchitis and infection are other indications.

Carbo vegetabilis (Vegetable Charcoal)

An important remedy for chronic digestive problems with flatulence, pain, gaseous formation and considerable discomfort. Also for weakness and collapse or when the reserves have been run-down by prolonged illness with weight loss. Slowness, uncertainty and fear are typical psychological reactions.

Carboneum sulphuratum (Carbon Bisulphide)

A remedy for tremor, weakness and paralysis, also impotence. The eyes are affected with a variety of degenerative conditions including neuritis, central scotoma (an opaque visual area), retinitis. Also for chronic digestive problems with flatulence, pain and constipation.

Carcinosin

There are several different types of carcinosin nosode (see section), all prepared from different types of cancer tissue, researched and developed by Drs. W. Lees Templeton and Donald Foubister. The major forms available are:- Adeno stom. (liver, car sickness, cyclical vomiting, anxiety), Lung (bronchitis and asthma), Breast (mastitis), Bowel Co. (rectal and anal problems, e.g. prolapse), Scirrhinum (breast cancer and threadworm), Uterus (for dysmenorrhoea problems).
The general indications are:- a cafe au lait complexion, blue sclerotics (whites of the eye), multiple moles, slowness and apathy, mentally retarded, depression, fastidious obsessional attitudes, obstinacy, tension, tics and mannerisms. The patient is better for thunderstorms and dancing (compare *Sepia*), better or worse for sea

air. He adapts a knee-chest position for sleeping. There is a family history of cancer, diabetes, tuberculosis, pernicious anaemia. He craves fats, milk, eggs, salt.

Carduus marianus (St. Mary's Thistle)

One of the 'organ' (for specific areas of the body) remedies of Rademacher, targeting problems of spleen and liver disease, particularly jaundice or recurrent haemorrhages. This approach is more 'pathological' rather than based on the totality of the individual symptoms and is therefore not truly homoeopathic.

Care of the Remedies

The homoeopathic remedies should always be stored in a cool, dark medicine cupboard, preferably in a clean glass container not previously used to store either allopathic or homoeopathic remedies. The remedies must be kept away from strong-smelling perfumes or camphor which could neutralise the vitality of the potency and lead to ineffective results. They should not be handled but taken from the lid, as the remedy is impregnated on the outside layer of the tablet or pill.

Caries (dental)

The common tooth decay of adults or children with degeneration of the dental pulp due to infection. Excessive quantities of sweet foods, convenience eating and poor dieting as well as hereditary weakness contribute to the condition, with diet being the major causative factor. The excess intake of vitamins can also mobilise calcium from the teeth, causing a deficiency and undermining dental health.

REMEDIES
To prevent caries and improve the dental resistance, include:- *Calcarea carb., Calcarea fluor., Silicea.* Also consider the individual constitutional remedy.

Cataract

There is a gradual diminution of vision with increasing mistiness of sight. General health is not affected. It is often a condition of the elderly due to either ageing or occupation (e.g. exposure to excessive heat, or from micro-wave damage), also associated with diabetes. The optical lens gradually becomes thickened and increasingly opaque. A comprehensive study on the subject was written by Compton-Burnett (see section).
REMEDIES
Calcarea fluor., Natrum mur., Silicea, Sulphur.

Catarrh

There is an inflammatory thickening of the area affected involving the mucosal lining, causing an increased secretion of mucus which may be either clear, thick, or yellow-green in colour according to the degree of infection and inflammation. The commonest affected areas are usually the nasal passages and sinuses, but the inflammation may also involve other areas, e.g. the middle ear, eustachian tube, vagina, rectum, bladder.
REMEDIES
Bryonia the discharge is white or clear, with dryness and irritation of the area.
Kali carb. for those of flabby build, all symptoms aggravated by a dry atmosphere and central heating.
Pulsatilla for nasal catarrh and sinusitis. The discharge is variable in colour and consistency, worse for heat.

Causation of Illness

These are many and complex, but in nearly all cases there has been a preceding stress factor to undermine vital resistance energy. Hahnemann placed a great deal of weight on such underlying psychological elements which he called the 'mentals' and from the start always emphasised that the key to cure lies within the mind. Where there is a severe illness, it is common for the physician to find that the very deepest psychological elements of the personality have been shocked, disappointed or traumatised in some way, often months or years before the onset of the illness. The resilience of the patient is undermined to such an extent that disease can penetrate, develop and take root. It is essential for cure that such mental factors emerge during treatment and are effectively treated by homoeopathy. Until they have come to the surface, the cure is often incomplete.

Cellulitis

The accumulation of fluid in the soft tissues and lymphatics immediately beneath the skin. The area is often unsightly and pitted. When stretched there is a typical 'peau d'orange' effect. Usually it is most noticeable in the upper arm, thigh and buttock regions. Other supportive treatments include:- diet, massage and exercise.
REMEDIES
Apis, Natrum mur., Urtica.

Centesimal scale of dilution

The principle of diluting one drop of the remedy mother-substance in 99 drops of the diluent fluid in serial dilution to obtain the homoeopathic potency. The sixth dilution commonly used in the U.K. is this serial dilution repeated six times, to give a dilution of 10 -12 or one part in a billion.

Cerium oxalicum (Oxalate of Cerium)

First introduced by Sir James Simpson, it is a specific remedy for congestion of the stomach mucosa causing vomiting. It is especially useful for nausea of pregnancy and travel-sickness.

Chamomilla (Chamomile)

A remedy for pain, restlessness and irritability. It is indicated for the young child who is teething, often with catarrh, and once held, refuses to be put down. Insomnia, impatience, crying, hot forehead, sweating and fretful irritability are characteristic.

Chelidonium majus (Celandine)

A remedy with a special predisposition for liver and gall-bladder problems. Jaundice and pain are characteristic. The pain is of a bruised type, situated under the right shoulder blade or in the gall-bladder area with tenderness. Drowsiness and nausea are other common symptoms.

Chenopodium anthelminticum (Jerusalem Oak)

For right-sided 'stroke' with loss of consciousness and heavy snoring-like breathing. Pains occur beneath the right shoulder blade. Speech is typically lost.

Chininum sulphuricum (Quinine sulphate)

A remedy for painful periodic problems, particulary rheumatic or gouty pains. The spine is often tender to touch and worse for the least pressure. It is also a remedy for kidney infections (nephritis), the urine thick, containing blood, uric acid and protein. It is useful for chronic malarial problems with a typical afternoon ague of shivering weakness and a rise in temperature, usually at 3.00 p.m. Pains in the head or behind the eye, may be severe. Sudden loss of sight may occur. It is also indicated in Multiple Sclerosis.

Chloralum (Chloral Hydrate)

Indicated for urticaria, conjunctivitis, asthma and insomnia from an overactive mind (compare with *Lycopodium)*. Also for delirium and confusional states.

Cholecystitis

There is infection of the gall-bladder with pain and tenderness in the upper right abdomen. The condition may or may not be associated with gall-stones. Symptoms include colicky pain - often severe, a raised temperature. A bile-duct obstruction may cause jaundice with dark urine and pale stools.
REMEDIES
Chelidonium, Hepar sulph., Mag phos., Sulphur.

Cholera

The severe bacterial infective condition of the bowel causing severe diarrhoea and collapse. The disease is often epidemic involving large numbers of the population and in the past, much loss of life. There was a London outbreak in 1854 when treatment was more successful using homoeopathic treatments than by conventional methods. Symptoms are severe watery diarrhoea, collapse and shock with vomiting and cramp.
REMEDIES
Arsenicum alb. for diarrhoea and collapse.
Camphor for diarrhoea.
Cuprum met. for cramps.
Veratrum alb. for severe cases of shock and collapse.
Isolation and hospitalisation are essential whenever possible. The disease is endemic in many tropical and European countries. Cases still occasionally occur in Europe, associated with the speed of modern travel, famine, natural disasters and siege situations. Antibiotics are recommended and these can be combined with the homoeopathic approach.

Cholesterinum (Cholesterine)

Indicated for liver disease. Typical indications are:- persistent burning pain in the upper right abdominal area, gall-stones, jaundice. Combined with a low saturated fat diet and weight reduction, the remedy can help correct cholesterol and triglyceride levels.

Chorea (St. Vitus Dance)

This disease of unknown origin is much less common than two or three generations ago when it was particularly frequent in hysterical female adolescents. At times the illness reached epidemic proportions with bizarre behaviour and multiple tic-like movements in whole communities. It is now rare - replaced by other social illnesses as anorexia, chronic fatigue syndromes and drug abuse. In many ways, these are more dangerous.

REMEDIES

Hyoscyamus when there is destructive behaviour.
Natrum Mur. for the underlying emotional problems.
Pulsatilla where the basic temperament is acquiescent and tearful.
Stramonium when there is great excitement.
Ignatia and *Zincum met.,* should also be considered.

Chronic disease

Problems that are long-standing and recurrent over months or years. These present as well-recognisable patterns of physical and psychological symptoms. The obviously indicated remedy gives but temporary relief and is ultimately ineffective whatever potency is used. It is for these conditions that Hahnemann advocated the use of a nosode (see section), to effect a change in a blocked vital energy response. He developed his classical treatise on chronic disease (1828) and theory of miasms (see section), with especially psora being a prime factor in causing energy-stagnation. There has been a lot of disagreement and dispute as to the reality and value of the psora concept. But undoubtedly it is of enormous help in appraising chronic problems and how best to treat them whether one accepts or not the causation of psora as originating with suppression of the 'itch' or scabies. The Bach and Paterson (see section) bowel nosodes have proved to be of value in such conditions and are worthy of study in order to extend the range of the therapeutic spectrum.

Cicuta virosa (Water hemlock)

A remedy for a wide variety of violent spasms, fits and convulsions, the head, neck and spine displaced backwards. The pupils are dilated. It's main sphere of action is on the nervous system and for this reason it is helpful for epilepsy, meningitis and head injury. The patient is restless, moaning and groaning, often childish, confused or delirious. The skin is infected, with a yellowish crusty eczema, or isolated large spots discharging pus.

Cimicifuga racemosa (Black Snake Root)

Indicated for depression with agitation, maniac restlessness and excessive talking. There are many uterine problems with pain, irregular periods, also recurrent miscarriage at the third month and puerperal psychosis.

Cina (Worm Seed)

The important children's remedy. It is of particular value in treating threadworm, with irritability, fits, teeth grinding, nightmares, nose picking and nighttime anal irritation. A dry tickling cough in the mornings is often characteristic.

Cinnamonum (Cinnamon)

A remedy for haemorrhage - as with nose bleeds. Always worse for exertion. The remedy also helps certain hysterical problems with symptoms in the gastric area, persistent vomiting, weakness and bone pains.

Circulatory problems

In most cases the blood supply to the periphery, e.g. fingers, hands and feet is poor and they are cold on the warmest day, the fingers sometimes white or blue. Painful cramps also occur, the cause either hereditary or familial. In the elderly the cause may be due to hardening of the arteries (arteriosclerosis). Intermittent claudication is cramp in the calf muscles on effort and may occur in young adults associated with excessive cigarette smoking. Pain resembling angina, is relieved by rest and due to an insufficient blood supply to the local calf muscles.
REMEDIES
Agaricus, Baryta carb., Carbo veg., Hamamelis, Lycopodium, Silicea.

Cirrhosis of the Liver

Usually a chronic condition with inflammatory changes in the liver cells leading to degeneration and eventual fibrosis. The causes are many, but often toxic irritation of the liver leads to the breakdown of normal cell function and health. The most common causes are:- chronic alcoholism, due to the toxic action of alcohol on the liver cells and aggravated by the lack of essential vitamins in the diet. Toxic poisons, especially carbon tetrachloride used in dry cleaning may damage the liver.

Increasingly, cirrhosis is the result of a viral type B hepatitis, associated with a blood or hypodermic needle source of infection. Inflammation causes destruction of the liver cells or atrophy and fibrosis, undermining the essential functioning of the hepatic cells. It can occur as a side-effect of certain drug treatments e.g. anti-depressants. The underlying cause must be treated when possible during the acute phase. Hospitalisation may be required.

REMEDIES

Nux vomica, Phosphorus.

Clarke, John Henry. M.D. (1853-1931)

The Edinburgh trained eminent homoeopathic physician. Editor of *The Homoeopathic World,* Consultant at the Royal London Homoeopathic Hospital, President of the international congress (1906). Clarke made major contributions to the literature throughout his life. His output was prolific and many of his writings, particularly his *Dictionary of Practical Materia Medica* is the standard reference to date.

Major writings include:

1885 Prescriber
1890 Dictionary of Domestic Medicine
1892 Rheumatism and Sciatica
1893 Therapeutics of Serpent Poisons
1894 Diseases of Glands and Bones
1895 Diseases of Heart and Arteries
1896 Heart Repertory
1900 Dictionary of Practical Materia Medica
1904 Clinical Repertory
1904 Life and Work of James Compton Burnett
1905 Homoeopathy Explained
1906 Whooping Cough cured with Pertussis

1907 Thomas Skinner M.D.
1908 Radium as an internal Remedy
1909 Vital Economy
1915 Gunpowder as a war remedy
1923 Hahnemann and Paracelsus
1925 Constitutional Medicine
1928 Colds, hay-fever and Influenza

Claustrophobia

A psychological problem that may be acute or long-standing. There is usually underlying insecurity, which comes to the surface as irrational fears of confined spaces - especially of being shut-in an enclosed space or any situation where there is any obstacle to a quick retreat. There is profound fear of fainting, diarrhoea, collapse, weakness or a nervous breakdown, 'making a show'. Any sort of exhibition or drawing attention is feared, at the same time, it is often an underlying tendency.
REMEDIES
Aconitum, Argentum nit., Ignatia, Lachesis, Natrum mur.

Clematis erecta (Virgin's Bower)

Acts on the genito-urinary system and particularly useful for chronic gonorrhoeal infections. The flow of urine is slow and irritating, the urethra constricted. It is useful for urethral blockage or stricture due to an old gonorrhoeal problem. The testicle is also swollen, hard and painful (orchitis). Other symptoms indicating the remedy are insomnia and neuralgic pains.

Close, Stuart. M.D. (1860 -1929)

The American homoeopath who studied under Fincke and Wells, graduating 1885 from the New York College of Homoeopathy. He was founder of the Brooklyn Hahnemannian Union in 1896, Professor of Homoeopathic Philosophy at the New York Homoeopathic College 1909-13 and President of the International Homoeopathic Association 1906.
Major writings include:
The Genius of Homoeopathy
1924 Lectures and Essays on Homoeopathic Philosophy

Coccalgia

Pain in the coccyx, or 'tail' of the vertebral cord. Symptoms may be constant or intermittent and often follow a fall or trauma to the area. In others it is arthritic or of stress or unknown origin.
REMEDIES
Arnica, Hypericum, Rhus tox., Ruta, Symphytum.

Cocculus (Indian Cockle)

An important remedy for vertigo, nausea, dizziness and feeling light-headed. Depression is a feature and all symptoms are worse at period times. It helps nausea of pregnancy, travel sickness, hemi-paralysis (one side of the body). The periods are very painful and too early. There is a tendency to never stop talking and intolerance of tight-fitting clothing is often diagnostic (compare *Lachesis).*

Coffea cruda (Coffee)

The remedy for restlessness, agitation and insomnia with neuralgic pains of the teeth or head. Palpitations, a rapid heart beat, heartburn and indigestion, are other indications for this remedy. The mind is over-active, unable to relax, causing extreme sensitivity.

Coffee

Because coffee is an artificial stimulant and a plant poison acting on the cardiovascular and central nervous systems it is not recommended during homoeopathic treatment. The initial stimulant effect is quickly followed by one of tension and a 'strung out' effect followed by a 'low'. It is a drug of social addiction. During treatment intake should be avoided or lessened considerably as it tends to reduce the efficacy of the remedies. It is suspected as having a possible link with cancer formation, particularly of the pancreas, a tumour which has increased in frequency over the past twenty years. Research in the U.S. has now been statistically validated, linking coffee drinking with this type of cancer. Where there is a craving for coffee to an addictive degree with over-excitability, give *Coffea.* For irritability, *Nux vomica* is often indicated.

Cold Sore (Herpes simplex)

A localised painful infective area of either the upper or lower lip, associated with catarrh or the common cold. The cause is a localised viral infection of the Herpes Simplex type which is usually benign and clears up within a few 7-10 days. In rare cases there is a secondary infection and a boil or carbuncle develops.

REMEDIES
Natrum mur. for cold sores affecting the lower lip area.
Pulsatilla for cold sores of the upper lip.

Colic

Severe abdominal pain causes doubling-up in an attempt to find relief. The pain is the result of spasm of the intestinal smooth muscle, commonly due to irritation from an infection or dietary indiscretion. A stone may provoke renal or gall-bladder colic. The condition is usually relieved by heat and rest. Agitation and restlessness are common. When due to the passage of a stone in the bile duct or ureter, there may be pallor, collapse and shock due to the severity of the pain.
REMEDIES
Arnica for shock.
Chelidonium for biliary colic.
Colocynth for renal colic with shock.
Magnesium phos. for intestinal colic.

Colitis

Colitis may occur at all ages, from childhood onwards. There is inflammation and sometimes ulceration of the lining mucosal layer of the large bowel or colon, with the passage of fresh blood, mucus and diarrhoea. The whole area is inflamed and irritated - the cause unknown. There is often an underlying stress factor, with 'bottling up' of emotions, particularly anger or rage. There is a tendency to a rigid obsessional make-up, the emphasis on control, all feelings unhealthily pushed down and denied. Hospitalisation is needed for severe cases, although an operation can often be avoided by the correct homoeopathic approach.

REMEDIES

Arsenicum, China, Natrum mur., Phosphorus, Phosphoric acid, Podophyllum.

The Common Cold (Coryza)

A throat and nasal viral infection, common at all ages, especially in the winter months. There is an acute sore throat, nasal and sinus congestion, headache, cough, feeling unwell, usually with no rise in temperature. Mild depression and exhaustion may follow the attack. The usual causes are:- multiple contacts during an epidemic, stuffy travelling or office conditions, cold, damp, fatigue, holidays with excessive exposure to heat and sun, or psychological stress which has undermined resistance and vitality.

REMEDIES

Arsenicum alb. taken hourly when there is marked debility and weakness with exhaustion, burning pains, headache and diarrhoea.

Nux vomica where the appetite is affected with constipation, nausea and irritability.

Complaints (of the patient)

Complaints or symptoms are what the patient feels and experiences of their illness. This dis-ease is the key to homoeopathic prescribing and the basis of its individuality and accuracy. The symptoms are listed and systematised in the Repertory, the most complete being Kent's *Repertory* which is a detailed major reference volume linking symptoms, aggravations and ameliorating factors with individual remedies. It is very important that the patient reports every symptom however odd, bizarre or trivial, to his doctor.

Complications of Homoeopathic Treatment

There are no true complications of homoeopathy except those reactions which are part of cure. They may appear briefly as an aggravation of a previous state with apparent worsening of symptoms. This happens as the remedy interacts with the problem area and makes it more available to the process of cure. When an earlier illness has been suppressed or not properly treated, then former symptoms may reappear. Normally this is only a temporary phase of the treatment.

Concepts of Homoeopathy

These are based on the Law of Similarities or *'Similar Similibus Curentur'*. Let that which can provoke illness also cure it, or let 'like' be treated by 'like'. Use of the 'similar' remedy is the cornerstone of homoeopathy, matching the proving symptoms of the remedy or its known toxicology patterns to those of the patient. It is fundamental to Kentian traditions in homoeopathy that the single remedy is used in the highest potency, and not repeated as long as there is an improvement. Individualisation, is prescribing for the individual patient and his symptoms rather than for a disease-pattern.

Confusion (Mental)

The processes of clarity of thought, judgement and perception are clouded. Causes include:- drug side-effects, infection, organic brain disease, arteriosclerosis, senility and psychological factors.
REMEDIES
Aconite, Natrum mur., Opium, Sulphur, Stramonium.

Conium maculatum (Hemlock)

An ancient remedy used in homoeopathy for chronic lymphatic and glandular conditions, especially where there is fibrosis and hardening of the glands. Its action is a generalised one throughout the body but it acts especially on the uterus, reducing spasm. It is helpful for painful scanty periods and breast conditions with hardness and painless enlargement *(compare Bryonia).*

Conjunctivitis

Inflammation of the conjunctiva of the eye with redness, irritation, lachrymation, pain or discomfort. Causes are:- local irritation, infection, a foreign body e.g. an eyelash is a common cause.

REMEDIES

Euphrasia, Pulsatilla, Sulphur in the 6c potency and as a local eyebath, using one drop of the mother tincture in the eye-wash, gives soothing relief.

Constipation

There is lack or absence of the daily bowel evacuation. The cause is often due to faulty bowel-habits and training in childhood, a poor diet lacking in fibre and roughage, lack of exercise, refined food and the use of laxatives over years. These may have led to a complete loss of the natural bowel tone. Many people become over-anxious when constipated and do not give the bowel enough time to respond before rushing to take another laxative.

REMEDIES

Alumina there is minimal bowel action, often aluminium kitchen pans have been used for a long period.

Bryonia is valuable when there is absence of desire and the stools are small, dried and round, like sheep droppings.
Nux vomica is indicated when there is desire but no push or ability to expel the stool.
Opium is recommended for severe and absolute constipation without desire. Take added bran with breakfast commencing with a teaspoonful daily.

Constitutional prescribing

The homoeopathic remedy, which matches the temperament and physiological configurations of the total individual, is usually given in high potency. When correctly prescribed it stimulates a vital healing reaction and a liberating feeling of relief and well-being. A recurrent problem is often resolved by the 'constitutional' and it is one of the most important principles of homoeopathic prescribing.

Consultation guidelines for the patient

Relate all symptoms felt which cause complaint or discomfort - however trivial. Do not give the diagnosis or supposed one unless it is one feared, or specifically asked for. Give every detail of the problem including the time of onset and any known causes. Describe if the illness has occurred before at any time and if so, when and how. Give details of the progress of the illness, any new or recent symptoms, why you have come to see the doctor now and whether any homoeopathic remedies have been taken in the past and their results. Describe any factors which either ameliorate or aggravate the condition with details of previous medical treatments or operations, including antibiotics or steroids. Mention any factors which have caused a change in the subsequent pattern of the disease. Give details of family or hereditary diseases known, especially tuberculosis, cancer, diabetes. Try to give a general historical picture from birth onwards, with special areas of sensitivity or problem. Be natural and spontaneous with your doctor. If you are feeling anxious or uncomfortable - tell him at the time.

Convalescent Remedies

During convalescence, it is important to remember that reserves of vitality are inevitably low and any excessive fatigue or effort should be avoided - particularly during the early weeks. A relapse is usually caused by stress or strain, at a time which should be quiet, calm and consolidating reserves.

REMEDIES

Arnica for post-operative convalescence three times daily.

Cadmium Phos. for after-flu weakness and debility.

China is indicated for more severe weakness and exhaustion after a long, drawn-out and debilitating illness.

Ferrum met. when anaemia and pallor with shortness of breath is associated.

Kali phos. for weakness and lack of reserve after any illness.

Phytolacca Berry is a useful tonic after illness, taken as the mother tincture.

Staphysagria for the immediate period after surgery.

Cough

There is irritation of the upper respiratory tract. The most common causes are:- a viral cold, bronchitis, laryngitis, polyps, substernal goitre. The cough may be dry or moist depending upon the condition of the mucosal lining. Stress is a common factor, often causing a dry 'nervous' cough which gives a crumb of comfort in a new or unfamiliar settings.

REMEDIES

Bryonia for a dry cough, with a little white sputum.
Drosera where a cough is dry, explosive and repetitive.
Hydrastis when the phlegm is thick and roped.
Ipecacuanha there is a moist cough, rattling and loud.
Merc. Sol. when there is a yellow, infected phlegm.
Natrum mur. for a dry 'nervous' cough.
Natrum sulph. when associated with bronchitis and shortness of breath.
Pertussin when the cough causes retching or nausea.
Spongia for an irritating dry cough.
Sulphur if there is severe infection and pus formation.

Cowperthwaite, Allen Corson. M.D. (1849 - 1926)

The 19th century American homoeopath, born in New Jersey and graduate of the Hahnemann college of homoeopathy, Philadelphia in 1869. He was editor of *The North-Western Journal of Homoeopathy* (1889-91). Professor of Materia Medica and Diseases of Women in the University of Iowa, he was also President of the American Institute of Homoeopathy. He then left Iowa, to teach in Chicago and later at the San Francisco Hahnemann Medical College of the Pacific. He was a poet and author as well as a physician.

Major writings include:
1877 Science in therapeutics
1880 Elementary text-book of materia medica
1882 Text-book of Materia Medica
1888 Disorders of menstruation
1891 Textbook of materia medica and therapeutics
Textbook of Gynaecology

Cramps (Nocturnal)

These usually occur in the calves or sometimes the dorsum of the feet. The cause is unknown but many are of circulatory origin.
REMEDIES
Arsenicum indicated when they occur in the early hours - just after midnight and have a burning quality.
Cuprum arsenicum is one of the most useful remedies.
Kali carb. is of value when cramps wake from sleep at a later time, between 3-5 a.m.
Pulsatilla is indicated when cramps are caused by the heat of the bed.

Crataegus (Hawthorn Berry)

The valuable heart tonic, usually prescribed as the mother tincture and taken in water. The main physical indications are:- palpitations, irregularity of beat, raised blood-pressure, breathless on exertion, heart failure, sweating. The principle psychological indications are :- exhaustion, depression and irritability.

Cravings (For foods)

These are often a manifestation of underlying depression and anxiety, or related to addiction to certain foods. They are important because they often give the clue to remedies, e.g. chocolate craving - *Lycopodium*, salt - *Natrum mur.*, fats - *Sulphur.*

Croton Tiglium (Croton oil seeds)

For extreme intestinal irritation with colic and explosive watery diarrhoea is characteristic. There is also severe skin irritation with burning eczema, or inflammation, the area bright red and burning (compare *Belladonna).*

Crystallography

Using patterns of crystallisation, it is now possible to differentiate clearly mother tinctures of the remedies. Research in this area is giving encouraging results and it is hoped that physical differentiation of the individual spectrum-potencies will follow as techniques improve.

Cullen, Prof. William (1710 -)

The eminent eighteenth century physician who advocated treating patients with a single remedy. His best known work was *A Treatise of Materia Medica* published in 1790. When Hahnemann was translating this text into German, he found himself in total disagreement with Cullen on the gastric action of *China* or Quinine in the treatment of Malaria. Hahnemann began taking Cinchona bark (quinine) as a clinical experiment, quickly developing the clinical symptoms of malaria and the first homoeopathic 'proving'.

Cuprum Aceticum (Copper acetate)

One of the best remedies for cramps in the calves at night or spasms of colicky pains in the abdomen at night. Nocturnal asthma, hay fever. There are many chronic skin problems. Also indicated in psoriasis.

Cuprum Arsenitum (Copper arsenite)

A powerful remedy for chronic renal failure and uraemia with burning neuralgic pains, chilliness and cramping pains. Intense cold is a feature of the remedy also sweating, asthma and colic. Also for carbuncle.

Cure

For a true cure to occur, there must be freedom from symptoms and relief from illness or pathology, also a liberation of the basic vital energy of the person. Cure is often relief from crippling exhaustion and fatigue with no reserves. In addition, there should be a basic alteration in the patients attitudes, perspectives and aims, especially when in the past these have been blocked-off, or kept vague, with a negative approach to life. Without this, there is a risk of a further relapse. The higher potencies help correct distorted perception.

Cystitis

Infection of the bladder with a frequent desire to pass water, discomfort or burning pain and often urgency. The urine may be cloudy and strong-smelling.
REMEDIES
Cantharis, Causticum, Hepar sulph., Pyrogen, Sarsaparilla, Sulphur, Terebinthina.

D

Dangers of Homoeopathy

These are rare and uncommon and when properly prescribed, homoeopathy is safe, non-toxic, non-addictive and does not cause psychological dependence. It is basic to homoeopathy that as soon as there is improvement, the remedy should be stopped. If they are continued needlessly during the period of recovery, they can in some cases stimulate the reappearance of the original symptoms and make them chronic. Such ill-advised prolonged prescribing is not in keeping with homoeopathic principles. There is another area of caution concerning the remedy *Silicea,* a deep acting and a powerful treatment of encysted conditions. It should be used with caution and only in low potency when there is a history of T.B. This avoids any risk of a cyst being re-activated into renewed activity by stimulating the breakdown of scar-tissue and drainage of residual infection or pus. Although the risks are slight, this confirms the importance of a thorough knowledge of homoeopathic principles and the past medical history of every patient.

'Dead' Fingers (Raynaud's phenomena)

The common problem where the ends of the fingers become white and bloodless due to poor circulatory control. It is often familial and may occur equally in summer as well as winter, although it is always aggravated by cold. The condition is not dangerous to health, unless very severe when tissue damage and ulceration may occur. The latter is rare however (Raynaud's disease).

REMEDIES
Hamamelis, Silicea. Where *Silicea* is not sufficient to stimulate a response, *Agaricus* or *Carbo veg.* may be required.

Decalcification

A general condition where the bones become transparent and more brittle causing osteoporosis (thinning of bone structure). The major causes are:- ageing with disuse of joints and hormonal imbalance. An excessive intake of certain vitamins, taken without caution over a prolonged period, may also cause calcium to be removed from bones and sometimes laid-down in other tissues to form a calculus. Trauma or infection, especially T.B. or osteomyelitis, are rarer other causes.
REMEDIES
Calcarea carb., Calcarea fluor.

Definition of Homoeopathy

Homoeopathy comes from the two Greek words *Homeos,* meaning equal or like and *Pathos* which is suffering or anguish. The basis of all homoeopathy is treatment using remedies which in their unprepared and otherwise toxic state, cause similar symptoms to those of the patient. Homoeopathy is a uniquely individual treatment using natural substances in their vitalised form, prepared by a process of dilution to stimulate the curative energies inherent within each individual. Increasing the dilution of the remedy substance, although lessening its material content, paradoxically increases its strength and power and deepens its action. The remedy must however be well-prescribed to be effective and match the overall picture of individual symptoms. The correct remedy is called the simillimum and is the underlying principle of *Similia Similibus Curentur* given to us by Paracelsus. The Latin inscription is best translated as 'let like be treated by like' - the cornerstone of homoeopathy and major treatment principle.

Delirium

A state of mental confusion, over-activity and hyper-excitability, usually associated with a high temperature or toxic state. There is wild delusional anxiety, disorientation, fear and restless, sometimes violent behaviour.
REMEDIES
Belladonna, Croton tig., Hyoscyamus, or *Stramonium.*

Depression

The familiar state of diminished spirits, with flatness, sadness disinterest and lack of energy. Various physical symptoms may be associated, for example chronic back pain or exhaustion. Any complaint that is not responding to treatment and is recurrent, may hide a depressive illness. The causes are many and varied, but include a physical shock to the system as miscarriage or childbirth, 'flu, glandular fever. In most cases there is an underlying psychological cause - either recent or remote, which was traumatic and led to feelings of rejection, loneliness, sadness or failure. Mourning and loss are well-known factors in depression and these can often recur, triggered-off by any event that recalls suppressed emotions, which were often denied at the time.

REMEDIES

Argentum nit., Aurum Met., Gelsemium, Ignatia, Lycopodium, Natrum mur., Pulsatilla, Sepia.

Dewey, Willis A. M.D. (1858-1938)

The eminent American homoeopath, graduate of the New York College of Homoeopathy 1880, Professor of Materia Medica and Therapeutics, University of Michigan. He also taught at the San Francisco Hahnemann College and co-authored several books with Dr. William Boericke.

Major writings include:

Essentials of Homoeopathic Materia Medica

Essentials of Homoeopathic Therapeutics

The Twelve Tissue Remedies (1934, co-author)

Diagnosis by the homoeopathic physician

This is always based on the totality of symptoms and according to the individual's response to underlying causative factors and their effect on his intrinsic vital energy reserves. Diagnosis is made according to the remedy indicated by the overall pattern of symptoms, rather than any underlying pathology, which the homoeopath considers of secondary importance to a primary undermining of reserves and vitality. In homoeopathy, a problem is not named as 'arthritis' or 'sinusitis', but according to the indicated remedy, for example *Rhus tox.* or *Pulsatilla.*

Diarrhoea

Excessive and uncontrollable looseness of bowel action. The causes are usually infection, but it may be emotional in origin or associated with underlying constipation which is the real problem.

REMEDIES

Aconite when the diarrhoea is sudden and acute, the patient extremely restless and apprehensive.

Arsenicum the stool watery, the patient prostrated, restless and anxious.

China for attacks of watery-green stools as with infantile diarrhoea or food poisoning.

Podophyllum is a useful remedy when the patient has watery-yellow, painless stools.

Sulphur is indicated where the stools are offensive, green and slimy. *Veratrum alb.* is for diarrhoea when the patient is collapsing, the stools painful, watery, with nausea, vomiting, weakness and profuse sweating.

Diet during Homeopathic treatment

Extremes of any description should be avoided in order that vital energy be given maximum chance to recover and not be wasted, before being re-established, with a stronger resistance and bank of energy resources. The diet should be regular, light and simple, avoiding excesses of spices and flavouring or rich food. The intake of tobacco should be kept to a minimum as should also coffee and tea, the latter being best avoided altogether during treatment. Foods should be steamed or lightly cooked and vitamins should only be taken on medical recommendation. The contraceptive pill should be continued as before but any side-effects carefully noted. During homoeopathic treatment, avoid instant or frozen foods and those containing sodium glutamate, colorants or preservatives. Eat fresh but not over-cooked dishes. High-fibre raw foods are helpful, supporting elimination and regular bowel movement.

Digitalis (Foxglove)

Tincture of the leaves of the mature plant. Indications are collapse, with a slow weak pulse, palpitations, angina, pneumonia, asthma and urinary infection. Depression is common. The patient wants to be alone (compare *Lycopodium*). Also for prostate problems, liver congestion with nausea and lack of appetite.

Dilatation of the Stomach

There is distention with pain and discomfort of the upper abdomen and stomach region or epigastrium.
REMEDIES
Argentum nit. useful for more general flatulence and distention, associated with intolerance of heat.
Carbo veg. where most of the trouble is in the upper abdomen and stomach area.
Lycopodium indicated when the symptoms are right-sided and situated in the lower abdomen.

Dilution of the remedies

This is the uniquely homoeopathic way of diluting the remedies. Using the decimal or centesimal scale and succussing, or violently agitating, the diluent each time it is 'reduced' in content, although the potency or strength of action is paradoxically increased. Succussing gives the remedy its unique homoeopathic properties and differentiates the remedy from a simple vaccine formed by dilution without dynamisation. The remedies are diluted by hand up to a thousandth dilution or M potency. For higher dilutions a machine is used to create the higher M and CM potencies. In general the lower dilutions of 6c act purely at a tissue level and the higher potencies on the mental or psychological processes as well as the tissues. But whatever the dilution, it is fundamental not to repeat the dosage or potency, once there has been an improvement.

Dioscorea villosa (Wild Yam)

Tincture of the fresh root, (first proved by Burt). Indicated for severe colicky pains of the stomach and bowel, also for biliary colic with restlessness and morning sickness of pregnancy. It is a remedy for severe pain, particularly of a neuralgic type. The main areas affected are the abdomen and bowel with sudden bouts of flatulence, colic and early morning diarrhoea, All symptoms are better for movement (compare *Sulphur)*.

Disease

In the homoeopath approach, disease is not seen in terms of invasion or infection, but as a primary disfunctioning or dis-ease, which has undermined the healthy process of vitality and resistance. Invasion or infection, with loss of functioning, are seen as much later secondary phenomena. In origin, dis-ease is either psychological or inherited and due to an underlying miasm undermining vitality. Stress is the commonest of present-day disease factors, leading to weakness and increased susceptibility to illness from the common cold, to a heart-attack.

Dosage

Dosage is not so important initially and only requires attention at a later date, when considering the level and depth of the primary causative disturbance. What matters most is that the remedy be prescribed on sound homoeopathic principles, according to the law of similitudes and not repeated once there has been a response. Certainly in the problem of chronic recurrent disease, higher potencies are often the only answer, sometimes in the 200c or M strength. The remedy will act in any potency or strength for the well-being of the patient and for this reason accuracy of the remedy is the main priority and dosage a secondary consideration, though nevertheless an important one for the physician.

Drosera rotundifolia (Sundew)

Tincture of the whole plant. Its main action is on the upper respiratory tract with a recurrent barking cough, nausea and vomiting. It is a very important remedy for Whooping cough. All symptoms are worse in bed, after midnight and from warmth. It has a role in the prophylaxis of Tuberculosis.

Drugs (prescribed)

Drugs are largely synthetic preparations, often used by the allopath to block or suppress the natural process of illness. The priority is always the alleviation of symptoms. Even the natural drugs of plant origin, such as digitalis, are now prepared synthetically and the naturally occurring alkaloids are lost to the patient in favour of more 'scientific' and convenient ones. The homoeopath will always put the needs of the patient before blanket-principles. Where a drug is required he will prescribe it, but in general he considers that most drugs are over-prescribed and suppress rather than stimulate a healthy response to the underlying condition. No form of suppression is used by the homoeopath unless pain or suffering is unbearable. The homoeopathic aim is a gentle stimulation of the fundamental well-being of the individual and powerful artificial remedies often oppose these fundamental principles.

Drysdale, John. M.D.

The Edinburgh graduate, and friend of Simpson, who settled in Liverpool and founded the Liverpool dispensary in 1837. There was a severe cholera outbreak in the city in 1849. As with the similar London outbreak, the results of homoeopathic treatment were outstanding and well below the corresponding allopathic figures with only 25.7% mortality. As a result of these statistics he was invited to apply for the post of physician to the city's children's hospital, but opposition was so considerable that he was forced to withdraw eventually. Co-editor of the *British Journal of Homoeopathy.*

Duboisia (Corkwood Elm)

A remedy which mainly acts on the nervous system. The pupils are dilated widely, the eyes painful and often irritated from conjunctivitis with red floaters (debris). Vision is clouded and restricted. Vertigo is common, the mind confused, foolish or vague. Insecure when walking,with a sensation of stepping into space.

Dulcamara (Woody Nightshade)

Prepared from fresh stems and leaves just before flowering. The 'barometer of remedies' with aggravation of all symptoms from any change of weather, but especially worse for cold or damp. Indicated for throat or chest infections, nasal catarrh, warts, hay fever, laryngitis with complete loss of voice. Summer diarrhoea.

Dunham, Carroll. M.D. (1828-1877)

The distinguished New York homoeopath. Qualifying in 1850, like Boenninghausen, he was converted to the homoeopathic approach following a dramatic personal cure, when conventional methods had failed. A friend of Constantine Hering (see section), he studied with Boenninghausen in Munster. An early advocate of the single remedy and the single dose, he later taught at the New York Homoeopathic Medical College and became President of the American Institute of Homeoeopathy in 1876. Translator of Boenninghausen and author of numerous review articles, he was also co-editor of *The American Homoeopathic Review.*

Dynamics of cure

This is the intrinsic energy of the patient, lost to him by the illness and a direct result of the basic disease, which lies beneath the more obvious symptoms. Homoeopathy is dynamic because the remedies have sufficient energy within them to overcome the blocks which shut-away and bind the patient's vitality. Freeing the patient's energy reserves by the power of the remedy, makes for a dynamic medicine and a dynamic cure.

Dysentery

Acute bacterial infective disease of the bowel, endemic in many tropical countries and marked by a high temperature, collapse, pain, the passage of watery diarrhoea, blood and mucus. It is especially dangerous to infants and the elderly.
REMEDIES
Aconite, Arsenicum, Sulphur for chronic cases. *Mercurius* for the acute symptoms.
Colocynth and *Nux vomica* for severe cramps.
When the case is at all severe, hospitalisation is recommended.

Dysentery Co (Bach)

The bowel nosode, developed by Bach and prepared from B.Dysenteriae. The main indication is extreme nervous tension with marked anticipatory anxiety (compare *Lycopodium).* Fear is marked, especially of new situations or strangers with shyness and fidgety restlessness. Palpitations, tics or involuntary movements of the face and neck, are common. Other indications are indigestion, flatulence and spasm, waking after midnight with acute pain, vomiting or colitis.

Dysmenorrhoea

The periods are painful and often irregular.
REMEDIES
Caulophyllum there are writhing generalised pains in abdomen and back.
Chamomilla the pains are severe, worse in the lower abdomen with irritability.
Nux vomica there is nausea, indigestion and irritability.

Pulsatilla for variable pains, tearfulness and intolerance of heat. Frequency of urination may be present.
Sepia the pains are very low down in the abdomen and have a dragging-down quality.
Veratrum alb. for menstrual colic with prostration and where bed-rest is essential during the spasms.

Dyspepsia

The common problem of indigestion, often due to over-indulgence or eating too quickly. Allergy or infection are other causes. The main symptoms are pain, flatulence, a sense of fullness, malaise with acidity and heartburn.
REMEDIES
Carbo veg., Nux vomica, Sulphur.

Dyspnoea

Difficulty and shortage of breath, either at rest or following the least effort. The causes are many but it is commonly associated with asthma, chronic emphysema, bronchitis, infection such as pneumonia, collapse of the lung, or cardiac malfunctioning with fluid on the lungs.
REMEDIES
For Asthma: *Arsenicum, Kali carb., Medorrhinum, Phosphorus.*
For Bronchitis: *Natrum sulph.* Where there is oedema, give *Antimonium tart., Arnica* or *Veratrum alb.*
For sudden collapse of lung (pneumothorax): give *Aconitum, Arnica, Phosphorus* according to symptoms, and hospitalise.

Dysuria

The condition of difficulty or hesitancy in passing water. It is commoner in men but may occur in either sex. The commonest causes are an enlarged prostate, infection, post-operative nerve-bruising, or after childbirth. It may also follow a lumbar-puncture and catheterisation.

REMEDIES

Causticum if post-operative or after delivery.

Hepar sulph., Cantharis, Causticum, Merc. sol., where the problem is of infective origin.

Natrum mur. for problems of nervous origin.

Sabal serrulata for prostate disease.

E

Ear ache

Usually due to infection of the outer chamber of the ear (external otitis), or the middle ear (otitis media). It is extremely painful with a high temperature and agitation.
REMEDIES
Aconitum in the acute and immediately painful phase.
Belladonna for heat, a red face and high temperature.
Mercurius there is a discharge of pus.
Pulsatilla pain is intermittent, worse for heat.
Sulphur for chronic or recurrent cases.

Early Diagnosis (importance of)

In every illness, as soon as the diagnosis can be made and treatment commenced, the better. Once a problem becomes chronic and long-standing, it takes longer to heal and the energy-reaction to cure is slow to respond and takes longer. For example, when a problem of psoriasis or eczema is treated in the early stages, a response is often rapid or immediate. But after several months, sometimes years of symptoms, the vital energy is exhausted and the patient depleted psychologically. Time must be allowed before a healing-reaction occurs.

Eating-out, fear of

This is a common psychological condition due to an underlying lack of confidence, which has become polarised to the area of putting food or drink into the mouth. The main symptom is tension when eating out in public, handling a cup or glass, and there is additional anxiety about any handshaking or tremor. It

can occur at any age and may only be of passing significance, although sometimes long-standing and a problem over many years. Other phobic anxieties may be associated, such as fear of crowds, claustrophobia and any situation without an obvious or easy exit.
REMEDIES
Argentum nit., Ignatia, Lycopodium, Pulsatilla, Sulphur.

Eczema

The common chronic skin ailment of infants and adults sometimes occurring from the earliest weeks of life. It is not advisable to suppress the condition using steroid ointments, as this may create a more chronic condition, just under the skin with little or no symptom-relief. The exact cause is not usually known but there is often an allergic factor present, or a familial tendency to the condition. It is quite common for one of the parents to have had a similar condition as a child. The commonest symptoms are redness and a slightly raised irritation, sometimes with cracks, oozing or bleeding, around the flexure areas of the limbs, wrists and hands. In severe cases, the whole of a limb can be swollen, the eczema bleeding from scratching, the child stiff with swelling, unable to sit down and crying with pain. There may be considerable flaking of the skin areas which falls like snow on the carpet.
REMEDIES
Apis, Belladonna, Graphites, Petroleum, Rhus tox., Sulphur.

Emotional Problems

The homoeopathic treatment of emotional problems is usually very effective giving a sense of well-being and confidence to the patient. This allows him to more clearly understand his feelings and motivations, as well as those of others in his psychological environment. All the major remedies contain an emotional sphere of action, and this can be used to the advantage of the patient.
REMEDIES
Argentum nit., Ignatia, Natrum mur., Lycopodium, Phosphorus, Pulsatilla, Sulphur.

Emphysema

The common chest condition with breathing difficulties. It is often follows many years of chronic bronchitis. The chest is fixed and barrel-shaped, breathing shallow and limited. The patient is quickly short of breath on effort, and susceptible to attacks of winter bronchitis.
REMEDIES
Ant. tart., Arsenicum, Hepar sulph., Influenzinum, Natrum Phos. Spongia, Sulphur, Tub.bov.

Epilepsy

The recurrent neurological illness, with fits or convulsions. These may be severe ('grand mal'), with loss of consciousness and bladder control, or the minor form ('petit mal'), with a temporary lapse of conscious awareness. The cause is usually of unknown origin although in some cases there has been a trauma, brain tumour, or infection in the past which has caused the condition. Treatment should be by an experienced physician. The patient often has a warning (an aura) of an imminent attack, which can sometimes be prevented at this stage, or precautions taken to minimise damage. Excessive coffee, alcohol, also fatigue, should be avoided.

REMEDIES

Aconitum, Arnica, Belladonna, Sulphur.

Equisetum (Scouring rush)

Tincture of the whole fresh plant. It is mainly indicated for bladder infection with irritation, frequency and cystitis, usually only passing small amounts of urine. The remedy helps pain in the bladder and kidney regions also bed-wetting. The bladder feels incompletely empty after passing urine.

Errors of prescribing

These are less important in homoeopathy than in other treatments because there are no side-effects of the homoeopathic remedy. Usually the wrong remedy simply fails to act or to elicit a response in the patient. Sometimes the patient is sensitive to a particular remedy which gives a very active response. This in itself is neither a danger nor undesirable, but it may cause anxiety and is best avoided in future treatments. A violent response to homoeopathy, either physical or psychological, is often the result of previous suppressant treatments, rather than the fault of the remedy. When this happens any remedy can quite simply be antidoted by its opposite or neutralised by giving *Sulphur* 6c three times daily.

Euonymus atropurpurea (Wahoo, Burning Bush)

A remedy for irritable confused states of mind. The liver and kidney areas are sore, due to congestion. There is a chronic gastritis, the stomach bloated, the abdomen uncomfortable and painful, with diarrhoea, the stools containing blood. Only small amounts of urine are passed. Fluid is retained, causing aching swollen ankles and feet.

Euonymus europea (Spindle Tree)

Prepared from a tincture of the fresh seed, the remedy is indicated for severe diarrhoea, cutting abdominal pains, chest pain with collapse and angina. It is essentially a left-sided remedy.

Eupatorium purpureum (Trumpet Weed, Gravel Root)

The remedy is prepared from tincture of the plant root. It is useful in bladder problems with irritation, incontinence, impotency, prostatic problems, uterine weakness, sterility. It is primarily a left-sided remedy, all symptoms are aggravated by movement.

Euphrasia officinalis (Eye Bright)

Prepared from tincture of the whole plant, it is mainly an eye remedy especially for conjunctivitis, inflammation, lachrymation, swelling of the lower eyelid with pain and intolerance of light. Also for hay fever, measles and irritation of the prostate.

Examination of the Patient

This is an essential part of homoeopathic procedure in order to make a diagnosis at every level. In homoeopathy the patient is primarily treated as an individual and this comes before all other considerations. Where there is a mechanical problem, this needs to be corrected - a narrowing due to scar-tissue needs dilating before homoeopathic treatment can work fully. A physical examination also confirms that homoeopathy is properly indicated and avoids the trap of unrealistic thinking that homoeopathy is a panacea for all illness. The need to exclude physical organic features is the major reason for making an examination in all cases. The homoeopathic doctor is foremost a physician and needs to look, touch, feel as well as listen i.e. the fundamentals of all good doctoring.

Examinations - fear of

This is the common 'funk' situation whenever there is a threat of something new and unfamiliar, or the possibility of failing to live up to high, unrealistic standards. This is often due to a conscience that is perfectionist, rigid and intolerant. An interview or examination situation is often over-valued, made too significant, or it lacks an overall perspective. The patient becomes paralysed by fear, usually of humiliation or failure. Homoeopathy is particularly effective for this type of problem and can lead to confidence and balance.
REMEDIES
Aconitum, Argentum nit., Gelsemium, Lycopodium.

Excitement and Elation

There are a variety of causes for this state of mind, varying from healthy youth and exhilaration, to drugs, alcohol, brain-damage, manic-depressive disease, or a high temperature. Most cases respond well to the indicated remedies which include *Aconitum, Belladonna, Hyoscyamus* and *Stramonium.*

Exhaustion

This is a common problem, seen increasingly in the young. The causes may be a physical, due to anaemia or chronic infection, the result of influenza, M.E., or post-viral fatigue syndrome, or following a prolonged debilitating diseases, such as hepatitis or glandular fever. Often there is no obvious cause to be found and the patient is depressed because of their lack of energy. Not uncommonly the reason is stress-related and lies with a pressurised lifestyle, lack of adequate sleep, regular exercise and fresh air. Other causes are:- a lack of overall plan or rhythm, or the body poisoned by over-refined convenience-foods which fail to give proper nourishment.

REMEDIES

Arnica is generally useful.

Arsenicum for acute cases.

China following an illness such as 'flu.

Kali carb. may be indicated in cases where anxiety is marked.

Kali phos. will boost energy, as long as the vital reserves are not completely exhausted.

But whatever remedy is given, the underlying cause must always be diagnosed and corrected.

Eye Problems

These vary enormously but respond well to the homoeopathic approach. Because the area is so specialised as well as delicate they are best treated by a physician with special experience in the area. The common problem of conjunctivitis responds well to *Euphrasia* or *Sulphur.* Styes are helped by *Pulsatilla,* an infection with *Mercurius. If the problem persists or is more severe, a specialist ophthalmic opinion is recommended.*

F

Faculty of Homoeopathy

The governing body of the homoeopathic physicians in the U.K., is based at the Royal London Homoeopathic Hospital. Many of its members are on the staff of the hospital. It governs the teaching, training and membership examination of the physician for the post-graduate homoeopathic degree following general medical qualification. The faculty is responsible for standards of practice in the country as well as for research, the publication of literature and information. It is linked with other countries and helps to organise national and international conferences representing the profession at all levels.

Failure to respond to the Homoeopathic treatment

There can be many reasons, but often it is because the patient is impatient and wants an immediate magical cure which does not exist. Homoeopathy is often slow but thorough, although in some cases the response to homoeopathy is rapid and dramatic. But this does not always happen and rapidity of response depends on many factors including:- the length of time the problem has been present, the amount and type of previous treatments and whether they have been designed to suppress or limit vital responses. Patients vary with the amount and quality of their intrinsic vital energy, sometimes a response is undermined by long periods of stress or a rigid diet which does not sustain it. Other factors are due to wrong prescribing - quite simply the correct remedy has not been given in the best potency for the particular individual. The remedy may also be inactive, or inadvertently neutralised and therefore ineffective. In other cases there is an underlying mechanical problem, a condition which creates a barrier to cure because of obstruction. A surgical or dental condition: - for example, an abscess that cannot drain naturally, must first be corrected by the most appropriate surgical drainage treatment before homoeopathy can give a positive reaction and a thrust towards health. Chronic disease due to miasmic factors was long regarded by Hahnemann as a cause of poor response to treatment in certain cases and this led to his theory of action of Miasms. Particularly Psora can lead to a weak or absent response, even where a remedy is well-indicated.

REMEDIES

Any underlying mechanical problem must be dealt with initially. Give *Sulphur* in the 30c potency, or the most appropriate Nosode.

Fainting (See section syncope)

Falls - cause and treatment of

These may be a simple accident of a healthy and inquisitive child, part of life's inevitable tumbles as a grown-up world is explored, or due to carelessness and inattention. In others they are part of being accident-prone (see section), and need special treatment and attention. In the elderly a fall is always serious and can lead to a fracture with immobilisation for weeks or months - the cause due to poor vision, sudden dizziness, weakness of limbs and movement, or confusion of mind.

REMEDIES
Arnica for shock and bruising.
Bellis perennis for tendon and muscle strain.
Rhus tox. for any strain.
Calcarea when due to weak ankles.
Kali carb. there is a tendency to accident proneness.
Lycopodium for general clumsiness.
Rhus tox. the cause is one of slowness and rheumatism, becoming off-balance.
Ruta when the vision is weak causing lack of awareness of obstacles.

Farrington, Ernest Albert. M.D. (1847-1885)

The eminent American homoeopath, physician and lecturer at the Hahnemann college, Philadelphia. Editor of Hering's *Condensed Materia medica*. He was an admirer of Swedenborg.
Major writings include:
1887 A Clinical Material Medica

Fasting - dangers of

A mild and temporary fast with fruit or vegetable juices, diluted with 50% spring water has much to commend it provided it is not continued more than two days and has been adequately prepared for (one or two days of raw foods). Similarly a fruit fast is also beneficial, provided it has been carefully considered and the system is not loaded with acid fruits which do not match the needs and constitution of the patient. A prolonged and more severe fast may also be both indicated and beneficial. It should only be undertaken under supervision and in conditions of rest and repose - in peaceful surroundings if possible. A major danger of a severe fast, is combining it with exposure to heat, especially the heat of mid-summer. It may cause extreme weakness and exhaustion of the vital cardiac energies to a dangerous level and lead to a severe anginal attack. This is particularly a risk where fasting is not medically indicated, or prolonged to a dangerous degree. The causes of recurrent fasting are often obsessional and psychological, with a distorted body image. See section on Anorexia Nervosa.

Fatigue (See section Exhaustion.)

Fear

Whenever fear is the predominant emotion which overwhelms a person, the remedy indicated is *Aconitum.* This is helpful whenever any condition has been precipitated by fear, even where it has occurred many years before.
REMEDIES
Argentum nit., Belladonna, Gelsemium, Lycopodium, Natrum mur.

Feet-restless

Fidgety or restless feet is often seen in an overactive child, nervous adolescent or an over-anxious elderly person, unable to relax. There is a tendency to be always on the move, doing something, up-and-down throughout the day. The cause may be stress-related, circulatory, senility or due to a drug side-effect.
REMEDIES
Arsenicum, Rhus tox., Zincum met.

Ferrum picricum (Ferrum picrate)

A useful remedy for stress-related conditions, especially when there are problems of over-activity with excessive pressure. An actor feels weak or collapses after too many performances without proper rest, or his voice becomes unreliable. It acts well in dark-complexioned people, when a well-indicated remedy has failed to achieve a cure. Frequency of urination at night, adds to fatigue. Also useful for prostate problems, including retention of urine. Warts are an indication, also corns.

Fever

The common condition of elevated temperature is usually due to underlying infection, but it may also be stress-related. Bed-rest is recommended with a fluids-only-diet, e.g. diluted fruit juices (grape or apple). Sponge-down until the temperature subsides. The cause must be ascertained in all cases and then treated.
REMEDIES
Aconitum, Arsenicum, Belladonna, Phytolacca.

Ferrum Metallicum (The metal Iron)

Trituration of the metal Iron. The principal indications are iron-deficiency anaemia with flushed cheeks, pallor, weakness, exhaustion, shortness of breath. There is irritability on the least exertion and allergy to eggs.

Ferrum phosphoricum (Ferric Phosphate of Iron)

Developed by Dr. W. Schuessler (see section). It is indicated for:- recurrent coughs and colds, anaemia, bronchitis, ear infections, laryngitis and rheumatism.

Fibroids

This is a simple muscle-cell tumour of the uterus, seen increasingly in young women. The cause is unknown, but thought to be associated with hormonal imbalance. They usually diminish in size after the menopause. When fibroids are large and cause pressure symptoms on the bladder, they are best dealt with surgically. In early cases, when the fibroids are small and not causing obstruction, give *Conium mac* three times daily.

Filix mas (Male fern)

Indicated for tapeworm. Constipation is a problem, also gnawing abdominal discomfort, often worse at night, with hiccup, colicky pains and itching of the anus and tip of the nose. The patient is pale and tired, with dark rings under his eyes.

Fincke, Bernhardt. M.D. (1821 - 1906)

A highly skilled clinician and graduate of the New York University school of Medicine in 1854. He was the first to potentise x-ray and President of the International Homoeopathic Association in 1896.

First Aid

Homoeopathy is one of the most effective forms of treatment for first-aid conditions of the home. Any bleeding must be stopped by local pressure, the wound cleaned with *Calendula* ointment or lotion. A foreign body must be removed - e.g. pieces of glass or splinter. Hospitalise to remove a foreign body if this cannot be done in the home. Give *Arnica* for shock, *Aconitum* where there is fear and restlessness. *Ledum* for small clean penetrating wounds. Where the wound is more red and swollen use *Apis.* If the area is red, hot and inflamed, give *Belladonna.* When there is weakness from loss of blood give *China.* If the patient is shocked and collapsed, keep warm in a blanket, with plenty of hot drinks. Give *Veratrum alb.* when pale, cold and collapsing. In all cases, haemorrhage and shock must be given priority treatment. If severe, use the Bach Rescue Remedy for shock, 5 drops every 15 minutes. Other remedies are:- *Arsenicum* for restlessness, *Hypericum* for lacerated wounds with pain shooting up the limb. If in doubt call your local doctor or hospitalise at once.

Fissure

This may be quite a deep crack in the tissue and resemble a fistula. It does not connect with any internal organ and a discharge is usually clear and due to local inflammation. The commonest site is an anal fissure when a split appears in the anal mucosal lining of the bowel, causing the most excruciating pain on bowel movement. There may be discharge of blood from the fissure onto the stools due to abrasion and irritation, or it may result in constipation from fear of a bowel movement. The stool must be kept softened by taking bran or olive oil in the diet for a few days and *Calendula* ointment should be applied twice daily to the area affected.
REMEDIES
Silicea.

Fistula

This is frequently a chronic condition with an irritating discharge, sometimes infected, from a tract which connects the skin or exterior of the body with one of the internal organs or the alimentary tract. It may be artificial and intentional, when carried out as part of a surgical procedure for drainage. When chronic the acute initial condition failed to heal for some reason. It may be due to trauma or infection, i.e. tuberculosis, the inflammation tracking down from an infected area to find a natural drainage point at the exterior. The latter is healthy and positive provided that the fistula heals and closes up subsequently and is not a constant cause of trouble and irritation.

As long as a fistula is still actively draining a condition, it should never be interfered with or surgically removed and stitched up. This can drive a disease-process deeper and create a more serious condition. One patient had a discharging fistula-in-ano excised surgically and closed. A year later she developed cancer. The link is not absolute or provable statistically, but the suspicion is sufficient to strongly advise non-intervention with what nature has provided. Drainage and free-flow of discharges from the body must in all cases be allowed without obstruction whenever they occur.

REMEDIES

Calcarea, Silicea, Tuberculinum, but do not use *Silicea* when the fistula is the result of an old T.B. condition.

Flatulence

The sensation of being bloated or over-full in the upper abdominal or epigastric area, also felt in the chest, and often due to the aerophagy habit of swallowing air. It is

common in children and sometimes adults. Flatulence is also provoked by eating rapid hurried meals, not chewed or properly digested and underlying stress.
REMEDIES
Argentum nit., Carbo veg., Lycopodium, Nux vom., Sulphur.

Fleury, Rudoph. M.D. (1903 - 1977)

The eminent contemporary Swiss homoeopath. Graduate of Zurich. Having studied in Paris and Vienna he settled in Berne and established his practice there. President of the Swiss Homoeopathic Society since 1950, and member of the International League. He is especially renowned for having introduced new methods in case-taking. Editor of *The World Directory of Homoeopathic Physicians* (1967).

'Flu

The common epidemic influenzal condition which can occur at any time of year and in any age-group. The symptoms are a raised temperature, prostration, aching pains in the limbs and joints, loss of appetite, sore throat, sinusitis, constipation or diarrhoea and depression. Treatment includes bed-rest during the febrile period, taking only liquids or diluted fruit-juices and as the condition improves, light, easily digestible meals. The condition is particularly dangerous to the very young and the elderly. Great care must be taken to avoid chest complications from premature exposure to cold or chill afterwards. For the very frail, antibiotics are often advisable, with homoeopathy in a secondary supportive role.

REMEDIES
Aconitum, Arsenicum, Gelsemium, Influenzinum, Nux vomica, Rhus tox. Use Cadmium phos. or *Kali phos.* during the convalescent period.

Fluoric acid (Hydro-fluoric Acid)

Prepared from Calcium Fluoride and Sulphuric Acid. It is a remedy for chronic infections, acting on bone and scar tissue, with a tendency to the formation of local infective areas. Whitlow, fistula, ulcers of the skin, varicose ulcers, fall within its range of activity.

Folliculinum

Also known as 'oestron', it is the natural hormone of the ovary. It has not been proved, but clinical experience has shown it to be effective for many female problems, especially at the menopause. The main indications are:- irritability; emotional instability; resentment, often about a restrictive or strict upbringing (Compare with *Staphysagria)*. It is also indicated for palpitations; weak or absent periods (use a low 3x potency), prolonged or heavy menstrual loss (use a higher 30c potency), vulvar pruritus (itching), a brownish loss between the periods, alopoecia of women, mastitis and fluid retention. All symptoms are worse before a period and after sleep.

Food Poisoning

This may be an acute non-specific infection of summer diarrhoea, or due to *Salmonella* food poisoning. The most vulnerable patient is always the small infant, because of the dangers of dehydration from severe vomiting or diarrhoea. When this is suspected, the child must be hospitalised immediately, having been given Rescue Remedy (5 drops) before the ambulance arrives. The main symptoms are vomiting and diarrhoea, with fever, collapse and exhaustion. The attack may follow eating ice cream or 'suspect' food and involve the entire family.

REMEDIES

Aconitum, Arsenicum, China, Colocynthis, Podophyllum, Pulsatilla, Sulphur.

Formica Rufa (Red Ant)

Tincture of the crushed Red Ant. Valuable in rheumatic and gouty conditions with darting burning pains and headaches. Vagueness, lack of concentration and facial paralysis are other indications.

Fractures

These must be treated surgically in a specialised hospital unit. The remedy *Symphytum* supports healing, once fixing and re-alignment has been established. Use *Arnica* for shock or haemorrhage, both before and after orthopaedic treatment.

Fragaria (Wood strawberry)

This is specifically indicated for allergic reactions to eating strawberries, especially when they present as an acute urticaria skin condition. The area is usually red or swollen and this may also involve the tongue. The remedy also helps prevent the formation of:- dental tartar, gout, renal or gall-bladder calculi and chilblains.

Fraxinus Americana (White Ash)

Tincture of the bark. Introduced by Compton Burnett. Indicated for uterine prolapse and fibroids with bearing-down pains (compare *Sepia).*

Frigidity

The common female condition of aversion to the sexual act with inability to achieve orgasm. The cause is always psychological, the roots deep and complex. Aversion to coitus may be quite unconscious, the cause traumatic in one form or other. The problem needs to be talked about, made less of a threat involving fear and failure. Where there is an on-going relationship with trust and sharing, without pressure to reach an orgasm, then sexuality can be more relaxed and tensions eased as confidence develops. The whole emotional approach to life may need to be considered and the personality aspects looked at with understanding, sometimes over a period of time. In all cases the intensity of the symptom should be reduced by discussion and gentle persuasion.
REMEDIES
Aconitum, Natrum mur., Pulsatilla, Sepia, Silicea.

G

Gaertner (Bach)

The bowel nosode, complementary to *Lycopodium.* It is indicated for malnutrition and stunted growth and is of value for children, as well as for the elderly, especially when associated with emaciation and a malignant condition. Other indications are:- a pale face with blue eyes, freckles, and long black eyelashes. The mood is one of fidgety restlessness, irritable, hypersensitivity and overactivity. There are many colicky gastric problems associated with an inability to digest fats. It is indicated in Coeliac disease, chronic gastric irritation syndromes and threadworm. Also for rheumatic pains, poor circulation causing chilblains and anal itching (pruritus).

Gait - awkward

The person is clumsy and awkward, lacking a movement which is upright and easy. A common cause is rheumatism or arthritis, affecting the joints and limiting movement. Others are due to hereditary disease, trauma, following any severe or chronic condition of the limbs, or after a surgical intervention with shortening or fixation of a joint to lessen pain (arthrodesis). Psychological factors, linked to anxiety or hysteria, are other causative factors.
REMEDIES
Lycopodium, Natrum mur., Phosphorus, Rhus tox.

Ganglion

The common localised swelling of the wrist area, due to thickening of the tendon sheath, causing pain or discomfort. The cause is unknown, but they are often provoked by a trauma.
REMEDIES
Baryta carb., Benzoic ac., Rhus tox., Ruta.

Gastritis

Inflammation of the lining mucosal layer of the stomach. The commonest cause is infective, but it may be associated with peptic ulceration, or irritation from a foreign body swallowed by a child. Major symptoms are pain and discomfort in the stomach region, the pain colicky with flatulence, sometimes nausea or vomiting.
REMEDIES
Arsenicum, Belladonna, Magnesium phos., Nux vomica, Pulsatilla, Sulphur.

Gelsemium (Yellow Jasmine)

Tincture of the root-bark, first introduced by Dr. Edwin Hale (see section). It is indicated for general infections of the influenzal type with marked lassitude, tremors and rigors. There is an irritable state of mind:- with aching generalised pains, collapse, diarrhoea and vomiting. Also of value in hysteria, examination fear and stage-fright. It is one of the most valuable first-aid homoeopathic remedies.

Gentiana cruciata (Cross-leaved Gentian)

Tincture of the root, first proved by Dr. Watzke. Indications include acute infections, especially of the stomach and throat. Also for colic, vomiting with watery diarrhoea and hernia.

Gentiana lutea (Yellow gentian)

A tonic remedy for problems of recurrent gastritis. Typical symptoms include:- acidity and stomach discomfort, persistent nausea, vertigo, loss of appetite, colicky pains, distention of the upper abdominal region.

Gentry, William. M.D. (1836 -)

The 19th century American homeopath, who in later life became a charismatic Christian healer.
Major writings include:
1875 An answer to the question - What is Homoeopathy
(1900) The Concordance Repertory of the more characteristic symptoms of the Materia Medica (in six volumes)
The Rubrical and Regional text-book of Homoeopathic Materia Medica

Gingivitis

Painful inflammation of the gums, the area soft and red with a tendency to bleeding.
REMEDIES
Ac. nit., Hepar sulph., Merc. Sol., Silicea, Sulphur.

Glaucoma

The acute or chronic condition of raised intra-ocular pressure, causing pain and visual disturbance. The condition is a serious one that requires specialist ophthalmic treatment. The cause is often unknown.
REMEDIES
Gelsemium, Natrum mur., Ruta.

Glonoin (Nitro-glycerine)

First proved by Dr. C. Hering. The indications are:- sudden violent pulsating headaches with bursting throbbing pain, violent hot flushes, worse at night, drenching night sweats and fainting. All symptoms are worse for the least jarring movement (compare *Belladonna).* It is a useful remedy for sunstroke.

Glossitis

Inflammation of the tongue, due to infection, trauma or from eating food which is too hot. The tongue is sore, red and may be swollen. Eating and swallowing are painful and uncomfortable.
REMEDIES
Rhus tox. the area affected is the tip of the tongue.
Arnica from trauma.
Apis for swelling of the tongue.
Ac. nit. there is blistering on the sides of the tongue.
Natrum mur. following a bee sting. (Also give Apis.)

Gnaphalium (Everlasting flower, cud-weed)

A remedy for sciatic nerve irritation and lumbago, left or right-sided, worse at night. Numbness is also present, alternating with the pain. Also for persistent colicky diarrhoea, irritability and dysmenorrhoea.

Goitre

Swelling of the thyroid may be the result of glandular overactivity: - causing a toxic condition with loss of weight, tremor, protuberant eyeballs, with exhaustion, or it may be due to a simple goitre provoked by the lack of mineral Iodine in the diet. The toxic goitre is most serious needing urgent treatment. If situated beneath the sternum, it may provoke mechanical problems (in addition to any hormonal disturbance), due to pressure on the oesophagus and trachea (windpipe) causing difficulty in swallowing or shortness of breath.
REMEDIES
Natrum mur for toxic goitre.
Thyroidinum for single goitre or thyroid deficiency.

Gout

Inflammation of the proximal or first great toe joint. High levels of circulating uric acid forms crystals which tend to deposit in the particular joint area which is affected. Symptoms are excruciating pain, incapacity, swelling with redness and often irritability. The cause is usually over-rich living, with excesses of red meat, and game with alcohol.
REMEDIES
Aconitum, Belladonna, Colchicum, Nux vomica.

Graphites (Black pencil lead)

Trituration of black pencil lead. One of Hahnemann's most valuable and important anti-Psora remedies. It is particularly valuable for skin problems especially acne, psoriasis and eczema. The eruptions exude a clear, straw-coloured fluid, often behind the ears. It is indicated for:- an obese, chilly make-up with frequent nose-bleeds, itching and weakness. The personality is over-sensitive, especially to music, weeping easily, depressed and exhausted with colicky pains, mucous diarrhoea, loss of reserves and vigour.

Grauvogl, Edward Von. M.D. (1811-1877)

The 19th Century German homoeopath, who practised in Nuremburg.
Major writings include:
1870 Textbook of Homoeopathy
1879 The Homoeopathic Law of Similarities

Grief (effects of)

Suppressed grief is one of the most undermining and damaging of all psychological conditions. It not only contributes to depression, but also provokes reactions of guilt, loss of confidence, fatigue and a variety of recurrent physical conditions that are resistant to all treatments. Symptoms tend to recur yearly, especially at the time or date of the loss (anniversary reactions).
REMEDIES
Ignatia, Natrum mur.

Grimmer, Arthur Hill. M.D. (1874-1967)

The American homoeopath, pupil and secretary to Kent (see section) for many years, one of his 'inner circle'. A graduate of the Chicago Hahnemann Medical College and a gifted homoeopath, he knew of the homoeopathic method since childhood and his parents' medical chest. He initially practised in Chicago, working closely with Kent on the *Repertory.* Later he lived in Florida and taught at the American Foundation of Homoeopathy for many years.

Guaiacum (Gum resin of the Lignum Vitae tree)

An anti-psora remedy acting especially on fibrous tissue, joints and ligaments, also muscles and mucous membrane, causing contractions in the area with deformity (compare *Causticum).* It is useful in chronic gouty rheumatic conditions with tearing shooting pains, stiffness and limitation of movement. Aggravated from movement, heat or cold, and damp.

Guernsey, Henry Newell. M.D. (1817-1885)

Born in Vermont and graduate from the New York University in 1842, Guernsey practised mainly in Philadelphia. Member of the American Institute of Homoeopathy in 1846, he became Dean and Professor of obstetrics at the Hahnemann Medical College of Philadelphia in 1957. He was significant in the introduction of the high potencies.
Major writings include:
1965 Introductory Lectures on Obstetrics and Diseases of Women and Children.
1867 The Key-note system

1870 Uterine Haemorrhage
1870 The Treatment of Disordered Dentition
1870 The Homoeopathic Materia Medica
1887 Key-notes to the Materia Medica
1877 Ovarian Tumours
1882 Plain Talks on Avoided Subjects

Guernsey, William Jefferson. M.D. (1854-1935)

The American homoeopathic physician and author. Major writings include:
1879 The Travellers repertory and Family Advisor for the Homoeopathic Treatment of Acute Disease
1882 Haemorrhoids
1883 Desires and Aversions
1885 The Card Repertory
1889 Guernsey's Boenninghausen

Gumboils

The recurrent infection of the gums with boil formation. The cause is often obscure, but frequently associated with dental problems and root infections.
REMEDIES
Merc. sol., Phosphorus, Silicea, Sulphur.

Gutman, William. M.D.

The eminent homoeopath who for many years practised in New York. A graduate of Vienna, he was an enthusiastic supporter of clinical research and international provings. He was President of the American Institute of Homoeopathy and chairman of the Research Council of the International League.

H

Haehl, Richard. M.D. (1873-1932)

The eminent German homoeopathic physician from Stuttgart where he spent most of his working life. He graduated from the Hahnemann Medical College, Philadelphia in 1898 and was also a member of the Homoeopathic Central Society of Germany. Haehl is most known for his excellent and comprehensive 2-volume *Biography of Hahnemann.* From the year 1898, he collected all the letters, documents and papers he could, visiting relatives to compile a comprehensive background. He worked closely with Boenninghausen's (see section) wife, who was a foster-daughter of Melanie, Hahnemann's second wife. He retrieved the important sixth edition of the *Organon* (with its extensive footnotes), from Boeninghausen's heirs and brought it to William Boericke in California for publication, also writing the preface.

Haematuria (Blood in the urine)

This may be due to a variety of causes:- including trauma, infection, a wart or papilloma, irritation from a bladder stone, a growth. In most cases, it is of minor importance, but it must always be investigated by a physician and a diagnosis made of the cause and source of the bleeding.
REMEDIES
Cantharis, Hamamelis, Phosphorus.

Haemorrhoids (Piles)

The common condition of piles due to varicosities of the anal venous supply and associated with chronic constipation or following childbirth. Symptoms are mucus discharge, fresh blood on the stools, pain or irritation. A pile may sometimes enlarge and become external, painful to the extent of preventing sitting.
REMEDIES
Aesculus, Aloes, Hamamelis, Lachesis, Pulsatilla.

Hahnemann, Samuel. (1755-1843)

The founder and father of homoeopathy. Born in Meissen Germany, where his father and grandfather had worked as artist-painters to the porcelain industry. He was an outstanding scholar and scientist from an early age as well as a gifted linguist. His studies were varied in both Leipzig and Vienna which gave him a breadth of vision and a sensitivity. Together with his knowledge and admiration for the philosophical works of Paracelsus, this led to his eventual insights and discoveries. The principles of homoeopathy occurred by chance when Hahnemann was translating the works of William Cullen in 1790. He took some Cinchona bark - the active ingredient of Quinine and to his astonishment, being in good health, developed all the symptoms of an acute intermittent, malarial-type of febrile illness. From these chance beginnings, Hahnemann tested or 'proved' over 100 new remedies with his proving group of dedicated doctors as well as himself and family. This led into the Law of Similars or the principle of *Simila Similibus Curentur* - 'Let like be treated by like' which is the cornerstone of the method. He advocated that the remedy be taken in the smallest or single dosage for cure, the remedies to be prepared quite uniquely by a combination of serial dilution and succussion at every stage. His theory of vital energy is amply described in his classic treatise the *Organon.* A contemporary of Goethe and anticipating Jung by 100 years, like Freud, Hahnemann knew the significance of the psychological, as well as the importance of the seemingly paradoxical stimulant to cause a physiological response or reaction, which both Goethe and Jung advocated at different periods and in different ways. Beset by opposition and criticism at many periods of his life, Hahnemann remained a tireless researcher, physician and teacher.

Major writings include:

1793 Pharmaceutical dictionary

Materia Medica Pura

1810 The Organon, revised six times in as many editions

1828 Chronic disease, in four volumes

Appropriately and aptly on his Pierre Lachaise (Paris) tombstone are engraved in Latin - *Non Inutile Vixi* - I have not lived in vain.

Hair Problems

These are commonly seen in the surgery for many reasons including hair-loss (see section Alopecia), or because the hair is thin, lacks vitality, or is greasy. The hair is an extension of the outer layer of the skin and a reflection of the basic health of the individual. Its lustre, bounce and general health may be affected by any upset to the system - including nutritional, hormonal, psychological or infective causes. The health of the hair is inseparable from the health of the scalp and also reflects any imbalance which may be present.

REMEDIES
Arsenicum for premature greyness.
Bryonia for dry hair often patchy.
China for weakness of growth after a prolonged and weakening illness.
Lycopodium for premature hair loss.
Natrum mur. for hair loss due to tension and anxiety.
Silicea the hair is weak or brittle, splitting and lacking vigour.
Sulphur associated with an infected scalp.

Hale, Edwin Moses. (1829-1899)

The American 19th century homoeopath who graduated from Cleveland in 1859. He introduced a whole series of new and valuable remedies to homoeopathy. These include *Gelsemium, Hydrastis, Iberis, Lycopus, Passiflora, Phytolacca, Plantago.* Hale was Professor of the Hahnemann's college of Chicago.
Major writings include:
1875 Materia Medica of the New Remedies

Hamamelis (Witch Hazel)

A circulatory remedy with special action on the venous flow. Proved by Hering. It is extremely valuable in varicose conditions, haemorrhoids and phlebitis and conditions where there is stasis and congestion, pain or swelling. Also indicated for haemorrhages from piles, menopausal flooding and post-operative recovery.

Harmony

That aspect of man which is the basis of all relaxation and true health. It is the essence of the internal vital balance, which homoeopathy aims to restore and maintain, and includes harmony at both mental as well as physical levels. Its presence is largely dependent on an uninterrupted flow of vital energy. When this is blocked or not available (often from stress), disharmony occurs. The struggles of the organism to correct and balance itself are manifested externally as symptoms.

Hartmann, Franz. M.D. (1796-1853)

The early German Homoeopath, born in Delitsch. One of Hahnemann's 'provers union', the original group of physicians, including Stapf, who worked in the development of new remedies and the repertory. He worked mainly in Leipzig and remained one of Hahnemann's earliest disciples and friend.
Major writings include:
1841 Practical observations of some chief homoeopathic remedies
1847 Hartmann's theory of acute disease and homoeopathic treatment
1849 Hartmann's theory of chronic disease and homoeopathic treatment
1853 Diseases of children and their homoeopathic treatment

Hawkes, Alfred Edward. M.D. (1849-1919)

The Edinburgh graduate and homoeopathic physician, mainly of women's diseases. He worked most of his life in Liverpool where he was physician to the Hahnemann

Hospital. Introduced to homoeopathy by Dr. Arthur Clifton of Northampton, he was a tireless worker and active to the journals and societies.
Major writings include:
1913 Mucous colitis treated with isotonic seawater
1914 Notes on a case treated with Tuberculinum
1814 Gastric Ulcers
1916 Retroversion of the gravid uterus
Other papers were written on: the Heart, Addison's disease, Alcohol, Seborrhoea.

Headaches

The common condition of head pains, either periodic and starting on one side as migraine, or a more generalised headache which is vague and varies in position from one attack to the next. When they are recurrent, it is important to find the underlying cause. This can vary from overwork, poor light condition, inadequate air and ventilation (building sickness), to dietary excess or infection. Visual causes (where a change of glasses is needed), require a check-up by an optician. There are many psychological reasons for headaches. The attacks may also have commenced after a trauma or accident, often provoked by a whip-lash injury or a problem in the cervical vertebrae which may need correction. Another common cause is catarrh and recurrent sinusitis. In all cases a proper diagnosis and full investigation is required as part of the homoeopathic approach to rule-out any underlying pathology requiring surgery or an allopathic approach, rather than a homoeopathic one. The patient's needs always come first. Having made the diagnosis, the best treatment for the individual patient and his particular headache can then be considered.

REMEDIES
Aconitum for very acute painful attacks.
Coffea there is severe pain with restlessness. There has often been considerable abuse of coffee over the years.
Kali carb. the pain is more often left-sided, in the mornings or late evenings, 'drawing' in type, and aggravated by airless conditions.
Lycopodium the pain is mainly situated in the right temple region, worse in the afternoon between 4-8.00.
Nux vomica there is irritability and the headache follows a period of dietary indiscretion.
Pulsatilla the pain is variable and worse for heat.
Silicea the pain begins in the occipital region and radiates forwards over the skull.

Health

That subtle and harmonious condition which is the aim of the homoeopathic physician with freedom from pain and dis-ease. There is a sense of well-being and relaxation, both physically and psychologically.

Heat

Always to be avoided in excess, especially when in a fatigued or convalescent state. If there is intolerance of all forms of heat consider *Pulsatilla, Argentum nit.* or *Sulphur* as possible remedies. If craving heat and cold on the warmest day, consider *Arsenicum* or *Calcarea.*

Helmunth, William Tod. M.D. (1833 - 1902)

The early 19th century homoeopath, poet and surgeon who graduated from the Hahnemannian College in 1853

Helleborus niger (Christmas Rose)

Tincture of the fresh root, 'niger'-referring to its black colour. There is irritability with shooting headaches and inability to concentrate. Indicated for old or recent head injuries with headaches, personality changes, epilepsy or convulsions. Headache and giddiness are aggravated by movement and the least draught of cool air.

Hempel, Charles Julius. M.D. (1811-1879)

The eminent homoeopathic writer and physician of Prussian origin. He studied and travelled widely in Paris and elsewhere before finally settling in the U.S. in 1835 where he studied medicine. Co-editor of *The Homoeopathic Examiner* 1843-45, Professor of Materia Medica and Therapeutics at the Philadelphia Medical College, translator of some of Hahnemann's most important works into English.

Major writings include:

1845 A treatise on the use of Arnica in contusions, wounds and sprains

1846 The Homoeopathic domestic physician

1853 A complete repertory of the Homoeopathic Materia Medica

1854 Organon of specific homoeopathy

1859 A new and comprehensive system of Materia Medica and Therapeutics

1860 Homoeopathy, a principle of nature

1867 Lectures on Homoeopathy

1868 The new remedies

1874 The science of Homoeopathy

1880 Materia medica and Therapeutics

Henderson, William. M.D. (1811-1872)

The Edinburgh graduate and later Professor of pathology at the university of Edinburgh, who gained prominence by developing a rational and scientific status for homoeopathy by his brilliant attention to research and detail. He was disapproved of by many contemporaries because they considered he was trying to make homoeopathy popular, by emphasising physical signs and pathology, rather than an overall symptom-profile of the patient. He tried to develop remedies for certain illness-conditions like bronchitis and pneumonia and was supported in this pathological approach by Dr Richard Hughes (see section).
Major writings include:
Homoeopathy Fairly Represented - in reply to Simpson's (see section) *Homoeopathy - Misrepresented 1845 Homoeopathic practice.*

Hepar sulphuris calcareum (Sulphide of Calcium)

Prepared by burning the crushed oyster shell with flowers of sulphur. It is an ancient remedy, proved by Hahnemann and indicated for chronic gouty conditions. There is over-sensitivity to touch and cold air, with marked irritability and exhaustion. It is an excellent remedy for infection, especially of the upper respiratory tract, tonsils, larynx and bowels. Indicated for offensive purulent conditions and painful infections with foul-smelling discharges, diarrhoea and urinary infections.

Hepatitis

The acute viral infection, causing inflammation of the liver and often accompanied by jaundice. There are several forms of the disease. Viral type A, is usually a mild illness, caused by contaminated food or water. The virus occurs in the faeces of the carrier, is spread by droplets, kissing contact, or flies. There is an incubation period of 14 to 42 days and full recovery usually occurs after a few weeks. Viral type B hepatitis is a more severe and prolonged form of illness. It is caused by infected blood or serum and typically follows the use of a contaminated hypodermic needle, syringe, tattooing, or a blood transfusion. The incubation period varies from 6 to 26 weeks. A third type of viral hepatitis also exists (non-A, non-B). Chronic hepatitis is a prolonged form of the illness which may last for many months.
REMEDIES
Bryonia, Croton tig., Chelidonium, Hepar sulph., Phosphorus, Sulphur.

Hering, Dr. Constantine. (1800 - 1880)

The eminent pioneer of homoeopathy in the U.S.A. He began his career as an opponent of homoeopathy, but on trying the remedies and theories in practise, he became its most active and ardent supporter, both in Dresden and Philadelphia. He founded the North American Academy for the Homoeopathic Healing Arts in 1835, the Homoeopathic Medical College of Pennsylvania in 1848 and the Hahnemann Medical College of Philadelphia in 1867. Hering was instrumental in proving and introducing *Lachesis,* the Bushmaster snake remedy, into homoeopathy. His great literary achievement was *Guiding Symptoms* in 10 volumes.

Hering's Law

During the course of homoeopathic treatment, symptoms improve from above downwards; from the most vital to less vital organs; from most recent to earliest symptoms and in reverse order of appearance.

Hernia

This is best treated surgically rather than by a truss or support, because of the danger of strangulation, or cutting-off the blood supply to the intestine within the hernia. When surgery is not possible for reasons of general health or unavailability, then homoeopathy is indicated as the primary treatment.
REMEDIES
Calcarea, Lycopodium, Nux vomica.

Herpes (Genital)

Infection with the herpes virus is increasingly a cause of chronic problems involving mucous membrane of the eyes, throat and genital regions in particular. It can also invade surrounding skin areas, with outcrops of herpes vesicles in the active phase. It is highly infectious, affects both sexes and causes varied symptoms as sore throat, leucorrhoea, cystitis. The condition is usually sexually transmitted. The disease is resistant to most conventional treatments and chronic cases often occur.
REMEDIES
Graphites, Hepar sulph., Natrum mur., Nitric ac., Psorinum, Rhus tox., Sulphur.

Herpes Simplex (See section - Cold sore)

Herpes Zoster (Shingles)

The common infection of the elderly with a chicken-pox type of virus. Second attacks can occur, but these are not very common. Any nerve root may be involved in the infection, usually of the abdominal region but at times the spinal nerve roots of the skull, or the orbit, are invaded affecting vision. There is severe pain, irritation, itching, blistering and typical scarring. Healing may take several months for full recovery, with neuralgic pain. Homoeopathy acts very effectively.
REMEDIES
Natrum mur., Ranunculus bulb, Rhus tox.

Hiatus Hernia

The common condition of herniation involving part of the stomach into the chest cavity, alongside the oesophagus, because of weakness (either congenital or due to strain), or damage of the diaphragm muscle. The condition is not serious, but it can be the cause of much discomfort, pain and heart-burn, particularly on bending, or when there has been a change of posture. If severe, surgical repair of the weak area of the diaphragm may be required.
REMEDIES
Borax for discomfort or heartburn on bending forward. *Nux vomica* is often very helpful.

Hip Problems

These are usually either arthritic or traumatic, rarely infective in origin.
REMEDIES
Mercurius for infective conditions such as osteomyelitis.
Rhus tox. the condition is aggravated by cold or damp, and better for movement.
Ruta when symptoms are improved by humidity. It is one of the best large joint remedies.

Hippocrates (460-377 B.C.)

The famous Greek physician, born at Cos and father of modern medicine. He introduced the Hippocratic Oath and codes of medical ethics for all practising doctors. Over 2,000 years ago, Hippocrates was first to record the basic homoeopathic principle that 'like cures like'.

Homoeopathy

The system of medicine that treats the patient as an individual, in its approach to the totality of the person, not just treating symptoms in isolation as if they were external foreign things, unrelated to the psychology, constitutional and vital make-up of the person. Symptoms are regarded as a key part of health rather than of disease and seen as the healthy response to underlying dis-ease and an essential part of cure. This vital symptom-response, is supported by the homoeopathic remedies, given in minute quantities to encourage and stimulate the body's intrinsic and natural vital response. Most of the remedies are of plant, mineral or animal origin and have been 'proved' on healthy human volunteers. These give a profile of symptoms which can be matched by the homoeopath to those of the individual patient. The correct remedy is one which in its natural and usually toxic form, would stimulate a reaction similar to, one which is the object of treatment. Suppression and blockage of symptoms by any method is regarded as dangerous to the patient, pushing the true problem 'underground' and not really curing the underlying cause because the emphasis is on the complaint, and not the underlying reasons for it. Usually the homoeopathic remedy is given in a single dose, or when repeated, it is stopped as soon as there is marked improvement in the patient's well-being and symptom-response. Homoeopathy was founded by Hahnemann at the end of the 18th century in the face of enormous opposition, from the conventional medicine lobby, which accused it of being 'unscientific'. Such opposition continued until recent years. Now it is much more accepted by the establishment and has finally begun to gain recognition in universities and medical schools of Europe as a 'respectable' speciality. But the fight for recognition has been long and there are still echoes of it in a few quarters. Each year more and more medical men and women are being trained in homoeopathy, but the number of doctors is still insufficient as the demand increases by patients who want a viable, safe, alternative method of prevention and cure.

Hughes, Richard. M.D. (1836-1902)

The eminent scholar and homoeopathic physician, working at the London Homoeopathic Hospital, although mainly based in Brighton with Madden, where he was physician to the Brighton Homoeopathic Dispensary. Hughes met with many critics, particularly

because he was a 'low' potency prescriber and his insistence on taking into account the site of action of the disease, the organs affected, the causative factors and the evolution of symptoms during an illness. He had a brilliant mind and his healthy questioning of dogmatic attitudes earned him many enemies. His fault was that he tried to popularise homoeopathy by making it more allopathic, emphasising the physical and pathological, rather than overall individual symptoms, the modalities, and the individualisation of the method. By trying to make homoeopathy more 'scientific' and respectable he was in danger of undermining the whole approach. Henderson, Dudgeon and Hughes (see sections) were the other major advocates of low potency prescribing. This caused an enormous rift in the profession, particularly from his former friend John Clarke and they became bitter opponents.
Major writings include:
1881 Hahnemann as a medical philosopher
Knowledge of the physician
Manual of Pharmaco-Dynamics
Manual of therapeutics
Principle and practice of Homoeopathy
1886 Cyclopedia of Drug Pathogenesy and repertory

Hydrastis canadensis (Golden seal)

Tincture of the fresh root, first proved by Edwin Hale and indicated in chronic catarrhal conditions where there is a discharge of thick, yellow, tenacious, sticky and stringy mucus. Reputedly of value as a prophylactic in pre-cancerous conditions and when there is a poor state of health, with vague symptoms of malaise.

Hyoscyamus niger (Henbane)

Tincture of the fresh plant. One of the major mental remedies for mental excitement with:- overactivity, delirium and delusional behaviour. The face is pale often twitching with emotion and irritability. There is intolerance to any form of covering although the patient is chilly. It is often used with *Belladonna* in treatments, but has less violence and redness.

Hypericum perforatum (St. John's Wort)

Tincture of the whole fresh plant, first proved by Mullen. One of the major first-aid remedies for lacerating wounds with lancing, tearing, stabbing pains shooting up the limb and sensitive to the least touch. Indicated where there is damage to nerve tissue, either bruised or severed, particularly of skin, nails, hands or feet.

Hysterical Problems

In this much-maligned disease, there is displacement of psychological energy into the physical, with the appearance of 'conversion' symptoms, which may be odd and bizarre, often resistant to all attempts to cure. The patient may be of any age, of either sex. Beneath the surface there are problems of security and sexuality, the latter seen only in infantile terms. Frequently there is an ambivalent attachment to one of the parents - never resolved since childhood. The hysterical disturbance tends unfortunately, to affect every aspect of living and relationships, with problems of frigidity, impotence, avoidance of the opposite sex, provocation and a tendency to be on display at all times. This helps compensate for feelings of inadequacy, at the same time making the most ordinary happening an 'event' and a cause for tension.

REMEDIES

Argentum nit., Gelsemium, Ignatia, Natrum mur., Pulsatilla.

I

Iberis (Bitter Candytuft)

Tincture of the seed, introduced by Dr Edwin Hale, as one of his new remedies. Primarily a cardiac remedy, it is of special value in angina where there is pain on effort, palpitations and distress. Vertigo with nausea, asthma, Meniere's Disease are other indications.

Ignatia (St.Ignatius Bean)

Tincture of the bean, it is indicated for suppressed grief and loss reactions, the patient never well since a bereavement or shock. Anal cramps and spasms with haemorrhoids are common. The mental state is one of tearfulness, anxiety and often globus hystericus (sensation of a lump in the throat).

Immunity to Drugs

Immunity to modern drugs can now occur so rapidly by new and evolving strains of bacteria and viral organisms, that it takes them less time to become resistant than for the pharmaceutical industry to develop another more powerful antibiotic to try and destroy them. Hence the folly of developing more and more powerful drugs with massive prescribing, using a sledge-hammer approach, with the ever-present dangers of totally resistant new strains emerging; the super virus or bacteria. Infections such as Legionnaires Disease, with no known specific treatment, is but one example of the emergence of seemingly incurable conditions hitherto unknown. In many hospitals, the presence of highly virulent strains makes them some of the least healthy and most dangerous places in Britain, with severe infections occurring in an environment that should be the most safe and healthy. Some wards have had to be completely closed down every year for several weeks or months for just this reason. In homoeopathy such problems do not arise. There is not the obsession with developing more and more powerful remedies to the patient's cost in health. There is no danger of provoking new and more dangerous strains of organism in our environment, as the major emphasis is on improving the 'soil' or resistance of the patient to stress, whatever form it takes. Conservation of reserves and vital energy must be maintained at all costs, for health to be regained or preserved.

Impatience

One of the most severe and damaging problems of our present generation and society. Remedies 'in a hurry' where time seems to pass too slowly include:- *Aurum met., Lilium tig., Medorrhinum, Natrum mur., Nux vomica.* The opposite, where time passes too quickly and there is never enough of it, indicates *Cocculus.*

Impetigo

The severe skin infection:- with pus formation, infection, swelling, redness, pain, temperature and discomfort. It can occur typically in debilitated adults or children. Although less common than previously, it can still at times reach epidemic proportions and be highly infective.
REMEDIES
Arsenicum, Merc. sol., Sulphur.

Impotence

The common male sexual problem. The causes are complex and often obscure:- including hormonal, nutritional, toxic or allergic, drug side-effects, or degenerative causes in the elderly. But of all the possible causes, psychological factors usually play a major role because of its emotional nature and the associations of the problem. Like its female-equivalent, frigidity; any underlying psychological factors, must be allowed to come to the surface, explored and discussed with any distortions and apprehensions sympathetically understood. A true hormonal deficiency needs replacement therapy in addition to the homoeopathic approach.
REMEDIES
Agnus cast., Lycopodium, Natrum mur., Selenium.

Imbalance

Imbalance of the human organism at deepest level, manifesting as malaise, fatigue, and illness on the surface, is what the homoeopathic prescription aims to correct. Whenever there is imbalance, from any cause, vital energy fails to function and flow freely and is totally blocked or displaced, contributing to many patient-symptoms. With the correct homoeopathic remedy in potency, such imbalance and blockage can be slowly adjusted.

Incontinence

Lack of control of urinary flow often with loss of sphincter tone. The problem is a complex one. The cause may be traumatic after childbirth, or associated with uterine displacement or prolapse. Infection, or degenerative changes in the elderly, also provokes weakness of the sphincter muscles.

REMEDIES

Baryta carb., Causticum, Sabal serr., Sepia.

Indications for the Remedy

These are the totality of symptoms of the patient, the modalities or aggravating and ameliorating features, any precipitating causes or antecedents, such as vaccination, when the patient has never been well since that time.

Indigestion

One of the major illness-problems of our present society. In many cases, there is underlying stress. Meals taken are usually of poor quality, eaten quickly without adequate time or enjoyment, so that proper secretion of digestive juices fails to occur. Excessive acidity plays havoc with the stomach and duodenal lining. An acute infection with vomiting or diarrhoea may further complicate matters.

REMEDIES

Arsenicum, Carbo veg., Lycopodium, Natrum mur., Nux. vom., Ornithogalum.

Indigo (Indigo dye)

This remedy acts on the nervous system and for this reason it is of value in epilepsy. It is also used for whooping cough when associated with epistaxis (nose-bleeds) and for recurrent sneezing, which is not linked to an acute infection. The bladder is irritated with a continual desire to pass urine, also dizziness, nausea, and a sensation of a tight band around the forehead. The mood is one of sadness or restless irritation. Indigestion with wind and belching is common, also sciatica.

Individuality - the patient as an individual

The homoeopathic approach does not see the patient as a disease entity to be 'neutralised' or hammered by massive doses of modern drugs at all costs. Hahnemann considered that the patient was first of all a spirit, then a mind and only lastly a body; and that treatment must be directed at all three elements in order for cure to be complete. Only the homoeopathic remedy is uniquely active in all three layers.

Individualisation of the Homoeopathic Approach

A characteristic feature of homoeopathy is that the patient is not treated as a collection of problems and sickness symptoms. Each person is unique and different and expresses an underlying malaise or infection, even in an epidemic, in his unique individual way. Each requires a different remedy from the other as they present and experience their illness differently, with varying areas of emphasis, anxiety and severity. Even twins, with an apparently identical cold or sore throat, may have quite contrasting symptoms which indicate different prescriptions. This individualisation rather than a 'nuts and bolts' or 'in for service' approach characterises the homoeopathic emphasis from the first consultation onwards. It is the individual that matters and how best to he!p the person. Homoeopathy is about people first, their individual needs, feelings and ideals, even more than it is about principles and remedies.

Infinitesimal dosage of Homoeopathy

This is not the basis of homoeopathy although many wrongly see it as synonymous with the method. It was developed late in the history of homoeopathy, mainly in America and many years after Hahnemann and it is not essential to the homoeopathic principle - which is fundamentally based on the Law of Similitudes and prescribing the simillimum remedy on the basis of the patient's total symptoms. Even if the remedy was not diluted at all, provided that it is prescribed on the basis of treating 'like by like', it would still be homoeopathic. Hahnemann for many years used mother tinctures of the remedies, but obtained side-effects which concerned him. It was only then that he began to experiment with diluting the remedies. He found by chance that instead of reducing the action and effectiveness of the remedy, it was further increased, not only safer for the patient, but wider and deeper in action. This troubled Hahnemann for many years as he could not understand how a process of dilution could apparently be continued to infinity, provided it was succussed or vitalised and still give more power to the remedy. He himself stopped at the 30c potency for most of his remedies and it was left to the American school to develop the 200c and M potencies at a much later stage. (For further general comments see section on Scientific principles). It is important to be quite clear that the potencies higher than 12c, do not contain any material presence of mother substance in the diluent. Such dilutions, although unique to homoeopathy, are not the fundamental principle of the method and even Hahnemann had his doubts as to their validity and efficacy; especially of the very high potencies. In recent years their clinical value has been proved by their enormous value in chronic problems resistant to all other means and also in constitutional prescribing.

Influenza (See section 'Flu)

Influenzinum (The Nosode of 'Spanish' Influenza)

The extract of the 1918/19 epidemic. Use the 30th potency and repeat hourly in severe cases. It can also be used for the common cold or coryza, when the 30c potency should be taken three times a week. Symptoms are:- weakness, collapse, muscle and joint pains, sore throat, catarrh and cough. In an epidemic it can be given prophylactically, either to give full protection or a modified course of illness.

Insect Remedies

The major insect remedies are *Apis* (Bee), *Cantharis* (Spanish Fly), *Formica rufa* (Red Ant).

Insomnia

The common problem of lack of sleep from impaired natural sleep rhythm, often caused by abuse of sedative drugs over a period, which has eroded the natural rhythms. We all need sleep for rest and to survive and the underlying causes of insomnia must be clearly ascertained and corrected. The excessive use of addictive, dependency drugs must be removed so that sleep can again take on a natural pattern.

REMEDIES

Aconitum insomnia is due to or provoked by fear.

Arsenicum the person wakes just after midnight or in the early hours about 1.00 a.m.

Coffea caused by abuse of tea or coffee over a prolonged period.
Kali carb. the person wakes between 3.00 and 5.00 a.m., falling asleep exhausted just before the alarm rings.
Lycopodium there is difficulty in getting off to sleep because of an over-active mind and fear of the future.
Nux vomica from dietary causes and late ill-balanced meals.
Pulsatilla when insomnia is due to getting over-heated in bed and then feeling chilly, never really comfortable at any time or for that matter in any situation.

International League of Homoeopathy

The co-ordinating body, formed in 1925, which sets the international standards for homoeopathy throughout the world and organises the international congresses, acting as a liaising body for the whole of the profession. Representatives of each country meet regularly to maintain high standards and co-ordination of research. The present members of the council (1994) are:
Dr. H Maas (President), Dr. D Toledo (Gen. sec.), Dr. M Kanan (Asst Gen Sec.), Dr. S Chase (Vice President), Dr. W Nold (Treasurer), Dr. M Philianos (Pharmacy), Dr. J Imberechts (Education), Dr. J Gnaiger, Dr. C Kennedy, Dr. G Resch, Dr. Soler Medina, Mr. C Day (Veterinary), Dr. J Gamarra, Dr. M. Teedemann, Dr. A Rost (Odontology)

Iodium (the element of Iodine)

Iodine in tincture. Works best for dark-complexioned people where there is wasting and thinness of limbs. Also for chronic infections, stroke or arthritis and restless excitable states of mind. It is useful in pneumonia with shortness of breath and cough. Fatigue, weakness and faintness are other common indications.

Ipecacuanha (the Ipecac plant)

Tincture of the whole root. Nausea with profuse vomiting, salivation, disgust for food, depression are the major indications. Lung congestion is a marked feature, with a loud rattling loose cough and difficult breathing. The patient is often sitting-up, sometimes fighting for breath. Whooping cough, breathless from excess of fluid and mucus in the chest, cardiac failure, haemorrhage, threatened abortion, are the other major indications.

Iris versicolor (the Blue Flag)

Tincture of the fresh root, first introduced by Kitchen. An early North American Indian remedy, it acts primarily on the alimentary tract. Major indications are:- severe burning pains of the mouth and stomach, vomiting, diarrhoea, colic and right-sided migraine.

Iritis

Inflammation of the ocular iris. For any acute inflammatory infections of the eye which do not resolve rapidly always consult a specialist-practitioner in order to avoid the dangers of chronic problems developing and the risk of permanent damage to vision.
REMEDIES
Duboisia, Merc. sol., Rhus tox., Sulphur.

Irritability

The common temperamental problem. In some cases it is provoked by trauma or concussion with a change of personality, in others, an expression of underlying depression and feelings of inadequacy.

REMEDIES

Nux vomica, Chamomilla, Cina, Colocynth, Hepar sulph., Staphysagria.

'Itch' The

The 'Itch' or Psora, now most commonly seen as Psoriasis, is the common miasm first described by Hahnemann, as the major underlying hereditary cause of chronic disease in our modern society. See Psora section for greater detail.

J

Jahr, George Heinrich Gottleib. M.D. (1800-1875)

Born in Saxony, Jahr had a most eminent and successful medical career as a homoeopath, particularly associated with the spread and development of homoeopathic principles in Europe, perhaps secondary only in importance to Hahnemann himself. He qualified in Bonn, but worked for most of his life in France and the bulk of his extensive practise and writing was done in Paris. His output was prolific, sound and thoughtful.

Major writings include:
1836 Manual of Homoeopathic medicine (4 volumes)
1841 Jahr's new manual of Homoeopathic Practice
1839 Elementary notions of Homoeopathy
1845 Jahr's symptom codex (or digest of symptoms)
1850 A new Homoeopathic Pharmacopoeia
1850 Alphabetical Repertory of Skin Symptoms
1850 Jahr's clinical Guide and Pocket Repertory
1856 Nervous Derangements and Mental Disease
1856 The Homoeopathic Treatment of Female Disease
1868 The Venereal Diseases
1869 Forty Years of Practice

Jaundice

Abnormal accumulation of bile salts, particularly bilirubin in the blood stream, causing the characteristic yellow discolouration. The cause is blockage of the bile duct which normally discharges into the intestine and gives the characteristic colour to the stool (as from gall-stones), or the problem may be in the liver, due to cell-blockage as from infective hepatitis, or certain tropical diseases. In the young baby the cause may be

a high level of blood cells which are abnormally fragile, from sensitivity to an inherited Rhesus factor from one parent. Infantile jaundice is dealt with by exchange transfusion when necessary. If mild, it resolves spontaneously within a few days.
REMEDIES
Chelidonium, China, Cholesterinum, Sulphur.

Jealousy

The common emotional state based on insecurity and loss of confidence. There is obsessional fear of loss associated with possessiveness. The preoccupation is always the same:- another person is a threat because of their beauty, wealth, sexuality, position, success, youth, intelligence, or any attribute that they seem to have more of. At the same time, there is under-valuing of the self, impairing maturity, confidence and relaxation.
REMEDIES
Apis, Hyoscyamus, Lachesis, Natrum mur., Pulsatilla, Staphisagria.

Jenichen, Julius. (1787-1849)

The early German practitioner, researcher and horse handler. He first developed the concept of 'high' potencies (over 30c) and believed that succussion was more important than the dilution.

Jones, Samuel A. M.D.(1833 - 1911)

The 19th century homoeopathic physician and teacher. Major writings include:
The Grounds of a Homoeopath's Faith

Julien, Frederick Bennet. M.D.

The homoeopathic physician, trained in Cork who spent much of his active professional life on the staff of the Liverpool Hahnemann Hospital and dispensary since 1921. He died at the age of 65.

K

Kafka, Jakob D. M.D. (1809-1893)

The eminent early 19th-century German homoeopath and editor of the *Allgmeine Hom. Zeitung 1872.*

Kali arsenicum (Fowler's solution)

Indicated for chronic skin problems. The area affected is dry and itching, with a recurrent eczema. It may be scaly and thickened, as in psoriasis. Fissures and cracks occur with bleeding. Also for localised nodules or thickening of the skin. A remedy for skin cancer, the patient is typically restless and pale.

Kali bichromicum (Bichromate of Potassium)

First proved by Drysdale (see section) in 1844, it is one of the major polycrest remedies of value in conditions with stringy, yellow, mucoid-purulent discharges particularly of nose and throat or where localised 'small spot' pains occur. Ulceration of skin, bone or mucous membrane is an indication for the remedy, as too a sore throat, the sensation of a 'hair on the back of the tongue'. It is particularly indicated for obese, fair-haired people, lacking energy and vitality (compare *Pulsatilla).*

Kali bromatum (Potassium Bromide)

The major indications area:- restless depression with exhaustion, impotence, chronic acne, and menopausal flooding.

Kali carbonicum (Potassium Carbonate)

The polycrest remedy for restless anxiety, depression and fear of solitude. A left-sided remedy, it acts on mucous membrane of the throat and alimentary tract, with chronic catarrh. Also for indigestion with heartburn, stitch-like rheumatic pains, asthma and hay-fever. All symptoms are worse from 3-5.00 a.m.

Kali hydriodicum (Potassium Iodide)

For loss of weight with palpitations, nodular skin eruptions, ulcerative and offensive purulent discharges. Depression with anxiety is common and chest infections, including bronchitis, pneumonia and asthma.

Kali phosphoricum (Potassium Phosphate)

Introduced by Schuessler (see section) into homoeopathy and proved by Allen (see section). There is a nervous restless depression with weakness or paralysis and yellowish discharges. Tremor with numbness is a feature and it is particularly indicated after shock or convalescence. Amenorrhoea, laryngitis, insomnia, with craving for ice-cold drinks and foods, are the other prescribing features.

Kali sulphuricum (Potassium Sulphate)

Introduced by Schuessler (see section) and indicated for infected skin conditions with yellowish discharges such as erysipelas, chronic nasal and bronchial conditions with catarrhal discharges, measles, scarlet fever, rheumatism. All symptoms are better for fresh air and aggravated by heat.

Kalmia latifolia (N. American Laurel)

Tincture of the fresh leaves in flower and proved by Hering. A valuable right-sided remedy particularly for problems of severe facial pain and neuralgia. It also helps:- angina, palpitations, shingles, wandering rheumatic pains, spinal paralysis with weakness of legs and problems of balance. All symptoms are worse for cold, movement or touch.

Kent, James Tyler. M.D. (1849-1916)

Born in Woodhull, New York, Kent was certainly one of the most eminent of all American homoeopaths. He practised mainly in Philadelphia and St. Louis. An able teacher, he was Professor of materia medica at the Homoeopathic College of St. Louis from 1881-88. Professor of materia medica and Dean of the Postgraduate School of Homoeopathy, Philadelphia 1889-90. Professor of materia medica, Hering Medical School, Chicago 1903-1910. He was co-editor of the *Homoeopathic Courier St.Louis* 1881-82, member of the American Institute of Homoeopathy, the International Hahnemann Association and founder of the Society of Homoeopathians. Kent advocated the single remedy and waiting before all improvement had ceased before repeating the dosage or remedy. He was instrumental in encouraging high potency prescribing and proved many new remedies. He was a great teacher, and some of our greatest prescribers have studied under him, including Weir, Borland, Gibson-Miller, Fergie-Woods, (see sections). He did more than anyone to bring homoeopathy back from being popularised, lessened by polypharmacy, prescriptions based on pathology alone. He advocated strict Hahnemann studies. For chronic problems, he advocated the 200c potency or above. Major writings include:

1897 Repertory of Homoeopathic Materia Medica - his greatest contribution

1900 Homoeopathic Philosophy - a fundamental statement of homoeopathic principles

1905 Lectures on Homoeopathic Materia Medica. This book is still widely used by students and practitioners and has become a classic reference volume.

Keratosis

The common condition of the skin, due either to ageing or excessive exposure to the sun over prolonged periods. There are small isolated greyish elevated areas, irregular in shape and unsightly, on either the backs of the hands or face. They are of cosmetic importance only, rather than of medical significance, or a cause of discomfort.

REMEDIES

Antimonium crud., Nitric ac., Sulphur.

Knee Problems

These are common at any age and in all cases a careful diagnosis must be made. Such problems are often arthritic or rheumatic in origin, but other causes as trauma, infection, sprain or degeneration must be excluded. The knee is swollen in acute rheumatism problem, either involving the knee alone, or as part of a more generalised inflammatory process. In the more simple and straightforward arthritic 'wear and tear' problems, there is less inflammation and heat locally although the swelling may be just as severe. Pain is common and can come from joints or the ligaments

with tear or strains being common. There may have been a fall with perhaps a fracture of the patella or tip of one of the long bones in the area. When in doubt an x-ray is essential.
REMEDIES
Apis, Pulsatilla, Rhus tox., Ruta, Sulphur, Symphytum.

Knerr, Calvin. M.D. (1847-1940)

The 19th Century American homoeopath and son-in-law of Hering.
Major writings include:
1878 *'Coup de Soleil'* - the homoeopathic treatment of Sunstroke
1896 Repertory of Hering's Guiding Symptoms
The Life of Hering.

Korsakow dilution

One of the earliest methods of serial dilution to produce the homoeopathic potency. It has been much more popular on the continent than in the U.K. The principle is to prepare the potencies by using the same recipient for each subsequent dilution, rather than a set of different glass tubes (Hahnemannian method). The Korsakow method assumes that in the centesimal dilution, when the container is emptied, one drop of dilution remains adhered to the surface of the container, so that the addition of 99 drops each time gives the correct c potency. It is still widely used on the continent as the K dilution and to prepare potencies above 30c. It is impractical to use separate vials at each stage of the higher dilutions. It is also used to prepare mechanically the higher potencies of 1M and above.

Kreosotum (Creosote in rectified spirits)

A valuable left-sided remedy for chronic infective conditions with purulent discharge, weakness and loss of weight. Also for chronic gum problems, tooth decay, irritation of bladder or prostate from infective causes. Chronic skin infections with irritation and discharging pus. The remedy can treat uterine infections with offensive discharges. A foul breath and tongue, vomiting, colic and an excessive canine appetite are typical symptoms of many psoric conditions and suggest the remedy.

L

Labyrinthitis

Acute infection or irritation of the inner ear, with severe giddiness, nausea, vomiting and exhaustion.
REMEDIES
Aconitum, Argentum nit., Cocculus, Conium, Cyclamen, Glonoin, Salicylic ac.

Lac Caninum (Bitch's Milk)

One of the most ancient medical remedies, introduced to homoeopathy by Reisig. It is of special value in diphtheria and severe sore throat. The pains alternate from one side to the other, with a bloody, purulent discharge, restlessness, anxiety and prostration. There are often fearful dreams and a phobia of snakes.

Lacerations

These should be cleaned with *calendula* lotion and any bleeding stopped by pressure, with all foreign material cleaned out and thoroughly removed. If severe, suturing may be necessary. Refer the problem to your family general practitioner or the casualty department of your local hospital.
REMEDIES
Apis for swelling and burning discomfort.
Arnica for bruising and shock.
Hypericum for nerve damage or bruising with shooting pains.
Ledum for small and clean penetrating wounds.
Ruta or *Bellis perennis* for sprains.
Phosphorus for bleeding or haemorrhage.

Lachesis (the Surukuku or Bushmaster Snake)

Introduced to homoeopathy and proved by Hering (see section), in one of the most dramatic and courageous of all proving. Typically all symptoms are worse from sleep, with intolerance of tight-clothing in any form and very sensitive to touch. It is a left-sided remedy having many uterine symptoms, including severe haemorrhage and flooding, also bladder or rectal infections.

Lachnantes (Red root)

A remedy for upper respiratory tract infections with:- sore throat, hoarseness, a dry cough, rheumatism of the neck region (with a stiff neck), rheumatism. (Compare *Causticum)*.

Lamasson, F. R. D. M.D. (1907-1975)

The eminent French homoeopathic physician and teacher, formerly a pupil of Pierre Schmidt of Geneva. He was President of the International League, the French Society of Homoeopathy and the National Institute of French Homoeopathy.

Lapis Albus (Calcium Silico-Fluoride)

Introduced to homoeopathy by Grauvogl (see section). There are burning pains in the stomach, uterus and breasts. It is of value in itchy skin conditions and reputed to have a role in the treatment of new growths.

Laryngitis

Acute or chronic infection or irritation of the laryngeal chords, with hoarseness, irritation and loss of voice. The condition may be emotional in origin with chord-paralysis until the underlying problem is resolved.
REMEDIES
Aconitum, Arum triph., Causticum, Dulcamara, Graphites, Hepar sulph. Sulphur. Chronic cases need careful diagnosis of the underlying causes.

Lassitude

The common condition of exhaustion with disinterest. The causes are many and include:- depression, anaemia, convalescence, fatigue from poor work and commuting conditions. It is indicated for chronic infection anywhere in the body, often associated with stress, a poor diet or fasting. Also before an acute physical illness has fully declared itself.
REMEDIES
Arnica, Arsenicum, Ferrum phos., Kali phos., Nux moschata, Sepia.

Laterality of the remedies

The natural predisposition of certain remedies to act more strongly and effectively on one side of the body than on the other.
Right-sided remedies include:-
Comocladia, Iris Versic., Kalmia, Lycopodium.
Left-sided remedies include:-
Euonymus, Kreosotum, Lachesis, Kali carb., Rhus tox.

Latrodectus Mactans (Black Widow Spider)

One of the most important spider remedies, using the tincture of the whole insect. Introduced to homoeopathy by Tafel and Jones. Its main indications are angina of effort, chest pain radiating down the arms, collapse and shock. There is a tendency to haemorrhage.

Laurocerasus (the common Cherry Laurel)

The fresh leaves contain prussic acid which give an indication of its potential toxicity in the undiluted state. It is helpful for:- chill, cyanosis, convulsions, collapse and lack of vital reaction. A cough is characteristic, with shortness of breath, clubbing of finger tips and cyanotic blueness, as occurs in certain cardiac or chronic lung problems. The cough is typically dry, spasmodic and irritating. The overall condition is one of weakness and near-collapse, the reserves minimal.

Law of Homoeopathic Cure

This is the basic law of the similitudes whereby, any natural substance able to create a physiological or psychological disturbance (when taken, by a healthy person), can cure similar symptoms in a sick person. It is traditionally summarised in latin by *Similia Similibus Curentur* or 'let like be treated by like'.

Laxatives

The amount of senna pods and other laxatives consumed by an average English family can be considerable. There is a desperate bid to stimulate natural peristalsis in a sluggish alimentary tract poisoned by over-refined foods, lack of exercise and roughage - made lazy by synthetic bowel stimulants. Often regular bowel habits and training have been absent for many years and causes both discomfort and anxiety. When used over a prolonged period, laxatives are undesirable and should be replaced by bran and particularly by foods rich in natural vegetable roughage. The avoidance of aluminium utensils in the kitchen is also basic. The appropriate homoeopathic remedy for this type of constipation should be taken until normal bowel action has been re-established and then stopped. In general, far too much energy and anxiety is centred around the problem, especially in the elderly and it should be allowed to resolve naturally without undue panic or urgency.

REMEDIES

Alumina, Bryonia, Nux vomica, Opium.

Lay Homoeopathy

The practise of homoeopathy by non-medically trained practitioners. This occurs now in several countries, including the U.K., although strictly outlawed in others as illegal medical practice. Training varies from a brief correspondence course to a three-year training and opinions vary considerably as to the advisability of the non-medical homoeopath. The B.M.A. set up a working party and inquiry to study alternative medicine and consider a possible Royal Commission. Now, over a quarter of qualified general practitioners in this country have had some experience of either receiving or prescribing alternatives like homoeopathy. In many cases where treatment is sought, the problem is not so much one of prescribing, but rather of making a diagnosis. Homoeopathy should not just be regarded as a panacea cure-for-all, or the inevitable prescription. Many cases require a surgical approach, or sometimes a combination of treatments including conventional ones and an antibiotic where vital energy is exhausted, or non-existent. The needs of the patient must at all times come before any necessity to prescribe, to treat, or prove a principle. There is much confusion in the public's mind concerning lay practice and the lay 'doctor' can undoubtedly pose a threat because of diagnostic incompetence, inexperience and lack of training. The lay practitioner must know his limitations and always work closely with a trained medically qualified practitioner and feel able to refer cases when in doubt. All qualified homoeopathic physicians are fully trained medical doctors. In all cases, diagnosis must be made at a proper pathological or disease level, as well as a homoeopathic one to ensure the patient's best interests. In Third World Countries, homoeopathy by the lay practitioner can be of enormous value and support to a local population and health programme, when working closely with the medical team. Its validity in other circumstances is often doubtful, the dangers for the patient sometimes outweighing the usefulness. A well-experienced lay-practitioner working in close contact with a doctor and part of a team can be of enormous value to a busy practice when no other homoeopath is available. A lay practitioner working in isolation with all the dangers of assumption and inadequate training can be a recipe for disaster. But a conventional doctor with rigid prescribing attitudes, refusing to take an overall appraisal of the patient, unwilling to ever consider an alternative approach to a problem, is scarcely better. In the U.K., the British Homoeopathic Association provides a list of medically qualified homoeopaths.

Ledum (Marsh tea, wild rosemary)

An important first-aid remedy which has anti-parasitic action. Weakness and coldness are typically present with lowered resistance. It is especially recommended for puncture wounds due to animal or insect bites as from a cat, monkey, needle-injury, bee or wasp sting. Redness with swelling and throbbing pain is an indication with chill and cold accompanying the inflammation or fever. In spite of general chilliness, all symptoms are worse for heat (Compare *Pulsatilla).*

Legs - heavy

Caused by poor circulation from leg-swelling and swollen ankles. The underlying cause is usually associated with varicose veins or infection, but sometimes the cause may be heart or kidney malfunctioning. In all cases the circulation is sluggish, fluid accumulates in the leg tissues causing discomfort.
REMEDIES
Alumina, Apis, Berberis, Carbo veg., Lachesis, Natrum mur, Pulsatilla, Rhus tox., Sulphur.

Leucorrhoea

The condition of white or clear discharge from the vagina which is often associated with irritation and frequently offensive. Causes are variable but include:- thrush, cervical ulceration, general fatigue and lack of reserves. Infection can also produce a thick discharge.
REMEDIES
Calcarea, Graphites. Kali carb., Pulsatilla, Sepia, Sulphur.

Libido

The innate sexual and ultimately vital energy of the individual. Its level of expression reaches a peak in adolescence, but it varies throughout life according to many complex factors, including psychological ones. The general level of health is reflected in a healthy libido. Absence or lack of libido can occur in conditions of:- infection, anxiety and depression, hormonal imbalance or deficiency, when taking the contraceptive 'pill' and often associated with fatigue. In all cases libido has a natural rhythm which varies with each individual and this must be understood by both members of a relationship in order to avoid misunderstanding and needless anxiety.

REMEDIES

For lack of libido consider *Kali iod., Onosmodium, Selenium.*

For excess libido consider *Belladonna, Murex, Platina.*

Lilienthal, Samuel. M.D. (1815-1891)

The American homoeopathic physician born in Munich who came from Germany in 1848. He qualified in New York becoming physician to the U.S. Homoeopathic Dispensary and Professor at the New York Homoeopathic Medical College and Hospital for Women for 20 years. He eventually settled in California where he taught at the Hahnemann College of the Pacific, with Dewey. Editor of the *North American Journal of Homoeopathy* (1870-85) and the *New York Journal of Homoeopathy* (1874).

Major writings include:

1876 Treatise of diseases of the skin

1878 Homoeopathic therapeutics

1886 Works on the materia medica
1886 Hereditary insanity
1887 Aetiology of tuberculosis

Lilium Tigrinum (The Tiger-Lily)

Tincture of the fresh plant and flowers, proved by Payne and Dunham (see section). The remedy has a powerful action on the emotions especially where there is restless depression or irritability. The basic make-up is often that of a martyr or 'do-gooder'. Pelvic symptoms are common, a bloated sensation, 'bearing down' pains *(compare Sepia)* and an offensive brownish leucorrhoea. It is also useful for angina pectoris. All symptoms are worse for consolation (compare *Natrum mur.).*

Lipoma

The small common fatty tumour, soft and mobile, which occurs in the skin at any age and for no obvious cause. They sometimes cause pain and discomfort, apart from being unsightly, stretching superficial nerves in an area of pressure or where friction occurs, e.g. the belt or bra-strap regions.
REMEDIES
Graphites, Pulsatilla, Sulphur.

Lippe, Dr. Adolph. M.D. (1812-1888)

The early homoeopathic researcher and practitioner who was a graduate of Allentown Homoeopathic College and one of Hering's earliest pupils. He was founder of the International Hahnemannian Association in 1880.
Major writings include:

Key to the Materia Medica
Textbook of Materia Medica
What is Homoeopathy?

Lips cracked

The common winter condition associated with painful chapping of face and hands.
REMEDIES
Arum triph., Bryonia, Graphites, Lachesis, Natrum mur., Silicea, Sulphur,

Locality of Symptom

This is important in the choice of remedy and may give the clue to prescribing, together with the overall assessment. For example:- pain in a small localised areas of the scalp (as if a nail is being driven through the head), is suggestive of *Thuja.* Pain just under the right shoulder blade or scapula indicates *Chelidonium,* for right-sided pain, consider *Lycopodium.*

Loneliness

This is a psychological condition which is increasingly common and similar to home-sickness often occurring after a change of environment or even a holiday.
REMEDIES
Eupatorium purp. or *Kali carb.* are of particular value for home-sickness.
Lycopodium is indicated for the person who feels lonely and insecure unless there is someone else in the house, although quite content to be in a room by themselves.
Pulsatilla feels lonely and insecure unless constantly surrounded by people to give reassurance and attention.

Lumbago

The common problem of low backache or pain, often incapacitating and paralysing and following a strain from lifting, poor posture, or exposure to damp and cold.

REMEDIES

Aconitum, Berberis, Bryonia, Nux vomica, Rhus tox.

Luna (Lactose crystals exposed to the moon's rays)

Indicated in illnesses influenced by the phases of the moon, particularly worms (as threadworm), or insomnia aggravated at the full moon. Also for certain psychological states, particularly lunar-excitement. Epilepsy and asthma may also be aggravated by the new moon. The remedy should be considered, where the moon influences or aggravates symptoms.

Lux, Wilhelm. (1776 - 1849)

One of the early homoeopaths and active in research. He was the first homoeopathic veterinary surgeon from Leipzig, developing the theory of Isopathy i.e. that every contagious disease contains within itself its own cure. Using infective materials he developed the first nosodes (see section) of Anthracinum (from Anthrax and Variolinum (from Smallpox).

Lycopodium (Club Moss)

Tincture of the Russian club-moss spores. Introduced by Hahnemann to homoeopathy, it is one of the most important of all polycrest remedies with powerful influence on emotional states of apprehension, fear and anticipatory anxiety as stage-fright, examination-fear and general insecurity. It acts strongly on the alimentary tract, especially for flatulence and indigestion. The lungs and bladder are supported and it is a valuable right-sided remedy, i.e. for right-sided pneumonia. It has a general tonic effect and is indicated for enuresis and is of considerable value in problems of impotence.

Lycopus (Bugle Weed)

Introduced by Hale (see section) as one of his new remedies to homoeopathy. Indicated whenever there are haemorrhagic tendencies, especially of the lungs or rectum, with shifting pains. The heart action is feeble and weak with frequent problems of palpitations and exhaustion. It is valuable in the treatment of raised blood-pressure.

Lyssin (Hydrophobinum)

The remedy prepared from saliva of the rabid-infected dog. Major indications are:- chronic headaches, excitement of the entire nervous system, pre-eclampsia (fluid retention, protein in the urine, a raised blood-pressure) of pregnancy, epilepsy and convulsions. The fits are worse for the sound of running water, or of water being poured.

M

Magnesia carbonica (Carbonate of Magnesium)

A major constituent of the notorious Gregory's Powder of the last century - used for acidity and constipation at the time. It is indicated in dark-haired constitutions, nervous and irritable, with marked exhaustion and prostration and oversensitivity to the least draught of cold air or touch. At the same time they are vulnerable, over-sensitive people. Alimentary problems also occur, especially colic with watery diarrhoea, vomiting and a sour taste in the mouth.

Magnesia phosphorica (Phosphate of Magnesia)

Introduced by Schuessler (see section) to homoeopathy and proved by Allen (see section). One of the major remedies for cramp and spasm with shooting, changing, bouts of pain. Cold air precipitates spasm or cramp. Better for heat and warmth, for bending, doubling-up. Often indicated in thin, anxious people, helpful for writer's cramp, also for exhaustion with sweating.

Magnesia sulphurica (Sulphate of Magnesia)

Collapse and prostration is severe with thirst and diarrhoea. The stools are thin and copious, frequently yellow and offensive. It is also useful for diabetes.

Manganum aceticum (acetate of Manganese)

First proved and introduced to homoeopathy by Hahnemann. Depression with irritability is characteristic, also anaemia. The skin has a bluish tint and chronic sore areas of ulceration, slow to heal. Every part of the body is over-sensitive and tender with loss of interest in food leading to increasing weakness.

Mania

The severe psychological disturbance marked by overactivity, talkativeness, insomnia, loss of judgement and insight, violence. It usually follows a severe depressive state, although this is not always in evidence or obvious. Nash (see section) recommended a triad of remedies:- *Belladonna, Hyoscyamus* and *Stramonium,* depending upon the degree of violence and activity in the manic state. Hospitalisation is often necessary.

Manic-Depressive States

The periodic psychotic illness marked by mood swings from the most profound and dangerous suicidal depressions to a 'high' excited states of optimism, agitation, insomnia and overactivity. The causes are usually obscure, but include inherited familial factors and instability in one form or other. Toxic poisons, infection, or psychological shock can also act as the precipitating trigger to manic-depression.
REMEDIES
Belladonna, Hyoscyamus, Natrum mur., Sepia, Stramonium.

Materia Medica

The homoeopathic materia medica is the total symptom-picture of each remedy, based on proving studies, toxicology, and clinical experience. Symptoms are grouped according to major physiological systems of the body e.g. lungs, heart, kidneys, etc., including the modalities and other distinguishing features which combine to form a total overall picture of the remedy's action. This data is then used to match the overall symptoms of the patient, confirming the homoeopathic indications to prescribe a particular remedy.

Mastitis

Inflammation of breast tissue, often occurring during lactation. It can also occur at any time from a blow or during a period of convalescence or debility.
REMEDIES
Aconitum, Arnica, Belladonna, Conium mac., Hepar sulph., Merc sol., Phytolacca.

Masturbation

Masturbation is not an illness or a disease, and should not be treated as such. It is a normal and universal expression of sexuality. In many cases its absence may be more significant than its occurrence. Only when painful or inappropriate, is there a possible cause for alarm or an indication for treatment, also when it becomes part of obsessional disease. In most cases it is the natural expression of our libidinal-tides and life-force. When it causes comment or problems the disturbance may be more in the commentator than the other person. It should not be made into an anxiety-laden 'heavy' area and a loving, tolerant attitude taken. It sometimes intrudes into an adult sexual relationships and undermines it, when counselling may be needed to explore any underlying causes. There are no specific remedies and any anxiety should be treated within the framework of the whole person.

M.E. (See section Myalgic encephalomyelitis)

Mechanism of action of homoeopathic remedies

The exact pathway of action of the remedies is still uncertain and a matter of research. The most likely mode of action is through the immune-defensive system using the natural antibody reactions to infection and stress. This has been confirmed by recent research studies using high potencies. The essential vital energy reaction (which is characteristic of the remedies) is canalised by the antigen-immune system, because the steroid group of drugs (which use the same pathway), inhibit the vital response or dampen it down. We also know that homoeopathy can act prophylactically or preventively in illness, where the correct remedies or appropriate nosode is used, suggesting a specific antibody pathway. Homoeopathy acts powerfully to lessen shock and severe stress reactions of trauma and accident which is again suggestive of the same immune mechanism. Doubtless we shall see confirmation of the exact mechanism within the next few years as research techniques improve.

Medicine - the homoeopathic system of

Homoeopathy is individualisation and contrasts with the allopathic method of treatment by opposites and largely based on synthetic products of the pharmaceutical industry. Homoeopathy acts in total contrast by gently supporting basic vital resistance and responses blocked by the disease-process. These vital responses are expressed by the healthy 'fighting reaction' of the individual and are basic to health and its maintenance. The key-point of all homoeopathic medicine is the use of the 'like' or simillimum remedy which produces similar symptoms to the patient's own reactions when in its undiluted form. The single remedy, unrepeated, is given as long as the patient is responding and is basic to the method. The principle of using small, serial dilutions, vitalised by succussion in the preparation of the remedy to avoid side-effects, is also characteristic of homoeopathy.

Medorrhinum (Gonorrhoea Nosode)

The medorrhinum nosode is prepared from gonorrhoeal-infected material. Major symptomatology is loss of memory and a sense of impatience, as if everything is happening too slowly, leading to impatient hurrying and irritability. Pain in joints is a frequent, problem and always worse in the mornings. There is a generalised tenderness, worse for touch and exhaustion. A painful tendo-achilles or ball of foot, is commonly present. All symptoms are better for sea air (compare *Natrum mur.).*

Medusa (Jelly-fish)

Indicated mainly for skin conditions with:- burning irritation, redness and blisters as in urticaria. Numbness. The whole area is swollen with severe discomfort. Anxiety is marked. Useful in allergic swelling of the face, lips and eyes.

Memory Weakness

In many cases this is due to stress so that concentration and attention is impaired, the memory not given a sufficiently concentrated stimulus for recall to occur.

Other causes are:- degeneration, fatigue, alcoholism or infection. During a convalescent period, attention is weak. After certain physical treatments as E.C.T. (electro-convulsion-therapy), the memory may be permanently impaired. In the majority of cases the cause is tension or stress, the memory weakness heightening any anxiety already present. When it is associated with aging, *Baryta carb.* is often helpful.
REMEDIES
Aurum met., Lycopodium. Lilium tig., Medorrhinum, Natrum mur., Nux vomica, Kali carb., Kali phos.

Menieres Disease

The degenerative condition of the middle ear with deafness, tinnitus, nausea and vomiting, or giddiness.
REMEDIES
Chininum sulph., Lycopodium, Salicylic ac., Silicea.

Meningitis

Inflammation of the meninges or fine membrane layer covering the brain and spinal cord and conveying the cerebro-spinal circulation and nutritional cushioning fluid. Most causes are of viral type in recent years, although the bacterial form can still occur. There is an acute infection, with irritation of the area affected. Symptoms include:- severe headache, high temperature, stiffness of the neck region, confusion, irritability, fits or delirium. Hospital treatment is recommended.
REMEDIES
Aconitum, Arsenicum, Hepar sulph., Sulphur.

Menopause - problems of

Because of an imbalance of oestrogen/progesterone hormonal levels, many distressing symptoms occur in the 40-50 year age group. It is primarily a female problem but symptoms also occur in the male. Hot drenching flushes, severe day and night sweats, irritability, tearfulness, tachycardia (rapid heart beat), anxiety, irregularity or cessation of the periods, and varying emotional moods, are the major problem areas.
REMEDIES
Calcarea, Lachesis, Lilium tig., Natrum mur., Pulsatilla, Sanguinaria, Sepia, Sulphur.

Mentals and Homoeopathy

The psychology of the individual and his state of mind has always been regarded as a key aspect of homoeopathic diagnosis and cure. One hundred years before Freud's genius gave us the importance of unconscious motivation and direction, Hahnemann firmly rooted homoeopathy in the psychology of the individual. The mentals or psychological aspects are given a great deal of attention in the consultation, especially any loss of drive, tendency towards depression, moodiness, or flatness of feelings. Excessive or unstable emotions, or anything that causes a flood of tears:- music, a book, film, dreams, also over-control, irritability and aggression, or the inability to express feelings, is important. Unreasonable fears, phobias or obsessional anxiety, the overall state of confidence and mental well-being are all as relevant as the physical side and specific symptoms - mental or physical. The mentals reflect the deepest and most important layers of personality. When a remedy is prescribed in sufficiently high potency it is often within these mental layers that a first improvement occurs:- a sense of well-being, feeling alive, no longer 'in gear' or 'driving with the brake on'. Even when there is a temporary aggravation of a physical problem at the outset of homoeopathy, the mentals often show the first improvement in attitude and confidence, and this is usually maintained as the patient improves.

Mercurius (Merc.sol., Quicksilver)

Originally the ammonium nitrate salt of the metal was used by Hahnemann, but in later years he used the trituration of the pure metal with superior results. This has been the practice since that time. Hahnemann both introduced and proved the metal as a remedy and gave a very comprehensive account of all its indications. Chilliness is common with profuse sweating. All symptoms are aggravated by both heat and cold and often worse at night. Offensive breath and sweating is marked with restlessness and tremor. Inflammation, ulceration with discharge of pus, is typical together with congestion of the liver, and tenderness over the area. Parkinsonism with severe tremor is another indication.

Mercurius corrosivus (Mercuric chloride)

This is an even more acute remedy than *Mercurius,* the symptoms very intense and violent. There are acute urinary symptoms:- with frequency, pain, haematuria and mucus in the urine. Urethritis with gonorrhoea or a greenish-yellow discharge of pus, is a common symptom. There may be an acute throat:- the tonsils ulcerated and discharging pus, an alimentary tract infection with diarrhoea, or dysentery-like symptoms.

Mercurius cyanatus (Mercuric cyanide)

Introduced by Beck for acute cases of diphtheria. The main indications are collapse:- the throat covered with a whitish-grey mucus thick coating, with rawness, difficult swallowing and painful speech. The patient is chilly and blue due to cyanosis from lack of oxygen. It may also be indicated as a prophylactic for diphtheria. (Compare *diphtherinum).*

Metal Remedies

It was the genius of Hahnemann that allowed the insoluble metals to be used in homoeopathic potency, by grinding them into sugar of milk until a soluble substance was obtained - called trituration. The major metal remedies are Copper *(Cuprum), Selenium,* Tin *(Stannum),* Aluminium *(Alumina),* Iron (*Ferrum),* Silver *(Argentum),* Gold *(Aurum).*

Mezereum (Daphne Mezereum)

Tincture of the bark taken before the plant flowers in February. There is a burning crusty eruption over the whole scalp or face with an itching eczema, ulcers and thick scabs, often whitish in colour. Everywhere there is a burning neuralgic-type pain. Depression is common with exhaustion and a peculiar (but characteristic) sensation of the teeth feeling too long. All symptoms are aggravated in the early spring when the plant is in flower. There is also aggravation from damp or cold and dislike of being touched or examined.

Miasms

One of the most important and unique contributions of homoeopathy to the treatment and causation of chronic disease. Hahnemann describes in *Chronic Disease* three major pathways of hereditary constitutional disease, containing not the disease itself, but its blueprint or 'shadow' of the original disease. Psora was most important or the 'Itch'. Sycosis is illness with a primarily gonorrhoeal root. Syphilis is the miasmic illness having a syphilitic origin in previous generations. Hahnemann worked for many years with his colleagues on the problem of chronic disease and developed a comprehensive list of recommended remedies for each miasm. For greater detail see headings listed under the individual miasm.

Migraine

The common syndrome of periodic headache, often one-sided, commonly beginning over one eye, associated with nausea, dislike of light and brightness of any kind. Prostration, flashing lights and sometimes vomiting as the headache becomes more severe and fixed, is characteristic. Migraine tends to occur in cycles with periods of several weeks free from all symptoms. Rarely, the typical migraine pains occur in the abdomen rather than in the head. It is often familial or related to food sensitivity, but in many cases, there is no clear pathological cause.

REMEDIES

Right-sided:

Coffea, Iris versic., Kalmia, Lycopodium.

Left-sided:

Kali carb., Lachesis. Also *Natrum mur., Silicea* .

Milk Allergy

Although this can occur throughout life, it is most commonly seen in the young child with projectile vomiting and failure to thrive, because of sensitivity to cow's milk.

REMEDIES

Aethusa, followed by a constitutional prescription.

Mineral Remedies

These form a large and most important group of remedies with far-reaching effects upon the patient, especially in:- areas of vitality, basic energy and energy-reserves as well as the internal health of the organs, alimentary tract and skin. Often insoluble, like the metals, they are made into soluble solution by grinding and dilution with lactose. They include *Silicea, Phosphorus, Sulphur, Antimony.* There are various very active mineral acids, for example:- *Fluoric acid, Nitric acid, Phosphoric acid, Sulphuric acid, Acetic acid, Benzoic acid, Oxalic acid,* as well as the various mineral salts as *Arsenicum alb., Magnesium phos.* Potassium salts include *Potassium carbonate, sulphate* and *bromide.* Sodium chloride in potency is the invaluable *Natrum mur.* another of the deepest and widely acting mineral salts.

Mixed Autumn Moulds (M.A.P.)

Tincture of three hay moulds - Mucor, Aspergillus and Penicillum. This is a most useful mixed homoeopathic preparation for hay-fever-like symptoms occurring in early autumn, particularly September:- with sneezing, nasal catarrh, tightness of chest, itchy eyes and throat.

Modalities of the patient

These are the characteristic constitutional features of the patient which are quite unique and relate to environmental responses to:- heat, cold, damp, wind, dryness, thunder, sea-air, water, heights, time of day, the season and foods. As a totality they create a sense of well-being, or fatigue and aggravation of the condition. For example *Pulsatilla* and *Argentum nit.* are both totally intolerant of heat in any form although *Pulsatilla* is at the same time chilly. In contrast *Rhus tox.*, *Arsenicum* and *Calcarea* all crave heat but in slightly different characteristic ways. It is the combination of the modalities combined with the total symptom-picture which makes for, the individualisation of the approach and accuracy of prescribing.

Morbillinum (The measles nosode)

Usually given in the 30c potency as a prophylactic treatment of acute, severe measles illness. Indications are:- cough, nasal and conjunctival congestion, sore throat, middle ear pain and involvement and the typical skin rash. In a very young baby it is of value when there has been exposure, particularly if the infant is weak, convalescent, or especially vulnerable.

Morgan Gaertner

The bowel nosode, prepared by Paterson (see section) from non-lactose fermenting organisms of the stool. It is indicated for:- pale, dark-haired, thin individuals with kidney, liver, and gall-bladder conditions, especially cholecystitis and renal colic associated with a kidney stone. All symptoms are worse in the late afternoon and early evening. Other indications are :- irritability and depression which may become suicidal in intensity, nasal catarrh, gastric irritability with heartburn, flatulence, constipation, leucorrhoea, asthma, psoriasis and insomnia.

Moschus (Musk Deer)

Tincture of the dried secretion of the preputial follicles of the Musk deer. The major indication is a tendency to faint easily, particularly at the least emotion, with pallor and chilliness. The patient looks deathly pale in the faint. Sweating and marble-whiteness adds to the general impression of lifelessness. It is useful in Pre-menstrual tension, but especially of value in nervous tension of the hysterical type.

Mother-tincture (symbol used is **θ**)

The basic remedy in solution before dilution. After agitation and thorough mixing, usually in a water-alcohol mixture, the mother-tincture forms the basis of the potencies. For the centesimal dilutions, one drop of tincture in 99 drops of the serial diluent fluid is used in alcohol solution. In some cases the remedy is given as the mother tincture, in drop form and not put up into potency, although prescribed according to simillimum principles. Here the remedy is needed to act at a strictly organ or tissue level only. The commonest example is *Crataegus,* taken as a heart tonic and commonly prescribed in this form as drops taken in water. Also *Phytolacca berry* for problems of obesity, *Sabal Serrulata* for prostatic problems and the remedy *Plantago.* But these are the exceptions rather than the rule in homoeopathy and for the majority of cases a potentised remedy is made up from the mother-tincture to encompass the mental side as well as the tissue level of the problem.

Murex (Purple Mollusc)

Trituration of the fresh juice of the shell-fish, first proved by Petroz. The remedy is indicated where there is:- hypersensitivity, excitement, emotional tension and hysterical tendencies, often with heightened libido. It is useful at the menopause when there are irregular periods with the formation of clots. There is a characteristic dislike of being touched or examined.

Muscle Pains

This is a common problem and treatment varies according to symptoms and cause. When traumatic in origin with bruising, *Arnica* is indicated followed by *Bellis per.* and then *Ruta* for injury to muscle. If the problem is rheumatic in origin with joint swelling or weakness, *Rhus tox.* is a major indicated remedy. When due to night-cramps of uncertain origin in the calf muscles give *Cuprum aceticum.* Pain in the calf muscles on exercise, may be circulatory in origin and require *Cactus,* but such symptoms are best treated under the direction of a physician. Pain associated with allergic swelling in the area may need *Urtica*.

Mutabile (Bach)

The bowel nosode, prepared from non-lactose fermenting organism, which mutates or changes on culture to become lactose-fermenting. It is indicated when there is constant changing or alteration of symptoms, i.e. when a skin condition such as eczema or urticaria alternates with a chest complaint, as asthma. It is also closely related to *Pulsatilla*, and this remedy is often required as part of the overall treatment.

Myalgic encephalomyelitis (M.E., Post- viral fatigue syndrome, P.V.F.S.)

This is a common fatigue syndrome. Although it may occur at any age, it is particularly common in young adults in their 20's. The main symptoms are:- an overwhelming sense of fatigue and exhaustion, blurred vision, variable numbness or cotton-wool sensations of the limbs, muscle weakness, aching or pain, feeling as if drugged or poisoned, with impaired concentration and retentive memory, anxiety or depression and often loss of confidence and panic. M.E. is a controversial illness, because it tends to follow a prolonged course over months or years and nothing specific can be found on physical examination or laboratory testing. The illness usually occurs after an acute viral influenzal illness:- of the throat, chest, or alimentary tract. For this reason it is also known as the post-viral fatigue syndrome (P.V.F.S.). M.E. has also been linked to severe allergic reactions to various food, including yeast and gluten, also to prescribed drugs.
REMEDIES
Arsenicum, China, the Glandular fever nosode, *Influenzinum, Kali phos., Nux moschata.*

Myxoedema

Deficiency of thyroid functioning due to simple goitre and lack of mineral iodine in the diet. In others, it is a complication of surgery for thyroid overactivity where excessive removal of thyroid tissue has occurred. Other causes are obscure and unknown, rarely of an infective or degenerative origin. In all cases, the cause of the underlying reduced functioning, must be ascertained and corrected.

REMEDIES

Baryta carb., Calcarea, Thyroidinum.

N

Naevus

The common pigmented beauty spot or mole. It requires no treatment unless very generalised or widespread and should not be removed or interfered with unless in a part of the body where there is constant irritation or they have changed in shape, size, thickness or surface form. In such cases they may require removal by an experienced surgeon.

REMEDIES

Carcinosin, Phosphorus, Thuja.

Naja (The Indian Cobra Venom)

One of the most ancient of all medical remedies using tincture of the fresh cobra venom. Many symptoms are of a cardiac nature with a burning, weight-like oppression in the chest and a slow pulse. There may also be cardiac collapse, the pulse slow, shortness of breath and a sensation of choking. The symptoms are aggravated by lying down and are usually left-sided. Depression is the commonest mental state.

Naphthalinum (Naphthalene)

Indicated for drowsy confusion and toxic infected states with delirium. Also for hay fever, whooping cough and threadworm.

Nasal Catarrh

The common often seasonal problem of inflammation and thickening of the nasal lining secretory layer or mucosa. There is congestion with discharge and infection. Catarrh may be allergic in origin and related to hay-fever particularly when it occurs in early June or July. The allergic response to the grass pollens causes irritation of the mucosal layer which accounts for the severe itching and watery discharge. A similar condition occurs in the autumn with allergy to late-summer tree moulds. Other common allergic substances are house-dust, foods, mites and animal hair. In others, air conditioning, over-heating and lack of humidity in the office, causes irritation and a chronic condition. A viral cold is a common cause of catarrh, the nose, throat and eyes affected by the inflammation. The temperature may be raised, with vitality and strength at zero, because of toxicity from the infection.

REMEDIES

Allium cepa, Gelsemium, Kali bich., Kali carb., Mixed pollens, M.A.P.

Nash, Eugene B. M.D. (1838 - 1917)

The highly respected and influential 19th century American homoeopathic physician, graduate of the Cleveland Homoeopathic Medical College (1874).

He was on the staff of the New York Homoeopathic College and President of the International Hahnemannian Association (1903).

Major writings include:

1898 *Leaders in Homoeopathic Therapeutics*

Leaders for the use of Sulphur

The Testimony of the Clinic

How to take the case
Leaders in Typhoid Fever
Regional Leaders

Natrum Carbonicum (Sodium Carbonate or 'soda')

First proved by Hahnemann and recommended for chronic psora conditions with severe skin problems of:- irritation, soreness, dry chapped burning hands and face without discharge. There is catarrh and a sore throat, the alimentary tract congested and causing problems of chronic indigestion. A similar problem occurs in the uterine area where congestion causes leucorrhoea. The predominant mood is one of depression and irritation, with twitching and exhaustion. All symptoms are worse for heat, music and effort.

Natrum Muriaticum (Sodium chloride or common salt)

One of the most valuable and important of all the polycrests and well-documented by Compton-Burnett (see section). Mental symptoms are:- depression with irritability, rigidity and tearfulness - worse for consolation and company. The remedy acts strongly on kidney functioning and has an important role to play in fluid and water balance. Retention, mental and physical, are a feature, fluid accumulating in the soft tissues of the body, especially the face, lower eyelids, which are puffy and bloated as the body generally. There is also chilliness and profound exhaustion, with a craving for excess salt in the diet. Chronic digestive problems and diarrhoea, are due to the sluggish congestion. Cataract may occur. Most symptoms are better or aggravated by sea air. *(Compare Medorrhinum).*

Natrum Phosphoricum (Phosphate of sodium)

Introduced first by Schuessler (see section) as a tissue-salt. A remedy for chronic problems of indigestion with sourness of taste or vomiting from excess milk in the diet. Lactic acid is usually in excess. The tongue is covered with a thick, sour-smelling coating and the diarrhoea is of a similar yellowish colour. Acidity, colic, flatulence and discomfort are marked. Depression with irritability is the predominant mental attitude, with general misery and dissatisfaction.

Natrum Sulphuricum (Sodium Sulphate)

Formerly 'Glauber's Salt' and first introduced to homoeopathy by Schuessler and Grauvogl (see sections). Primarily it is a remedy for sycotic conditions where the symptoms are in the pancreatic bile duct regions which are not functioning effectively. There is chronic indigestion, constipation, colic - the whole intestinal region tender and sluggish. Bladder problems are common with frequency, bed-wetting and constipation. All symptoms are worse for damp or cold, tight clothing, music and are better for cold dry weather and fresh air.

Nausea

The sensation of general malaise, sweating and weakness with an overwhelming desire to vomit. The condition may be provoked by a gastric upset following a dietary indiscretion or acute infection. It is also common in the early months of pregnancy. Many cases are psychological in origin and provide an exit from a threatening, overwhelming situation.

REMEDIES
Argentum nit., Cocculus, Ipecac., Natrum mur., Nux vomica, Petroleum, Pulsatilla.

Neatby, Edwin A. M.D. (1858-1933)

The London homoeopath and nephew of Thomas Neatby (see section), working in general practice with his uncle in Hampstead, before specialising in gynaecology. Eventually physician for diseases of women at the London Homoeopathic Hospital in 1922. President of the British Homoeopathic Society in 1897 and 1919, Founder of the Missionary School in 1903 and later Dean, establishing its premises at 2, Powis Place. He was responsible for much of the school's appeal and success. Author of many articles in the homoeopathic journals.
Major writings include:
A manual of Tropical Medicine and hygiene, (written with Thomas Miller Neatby)
A manual of homoeotherapeutics (written with T. Stonham)

Neatby, Thomas Miller. M.D.

One of the early homoeopathic physicians of the century, physician to the London Homoeopathic Hospital and the Missionary School. He was conservative in his approach, a pupil and active supporter of Hughes (see section) and his pathological approach and logic. He opposed the then new American ideas of high, single remedy prescriptions and potencies. He was co-author of *A Handbook of Tropical Medicine and Hygiene* with his nephew Edwin Neatby.

Neck pain and stiffness

The common problem of pain and aching discomfort in the neck area. The cause is variable - and may be from a simple traumatic cause with bruising and spasm, or exposure to a draught, with chilling and tension in local muscles of the area, also tenderness and stiffness. Muscular rheumatism is a more recurrent problem, related to damp or sudden climatic changes, aggravated by age and poor health. Neck pain may also come from a nearby vertebral cause where arthritis, displacement, infection, or any localised condition causes pressure or irritation. The condition may be acute or chronic. Not uncommonly it is psychological in origin, the tension and pain due to underlying anxiety and reflecting deeper problems. If more hysterical in type, symptoms can be incapacitating with a dramatic, attention-seeking element which defies all attempts at either diagnosis or cure.
REMEDIES
Aconitum, Arnica, Causticum, Natrum mur., Rhus tox., Sulphur.

Nephritis

Strictly pyelonephritis with infection of the kidney tissue. Common in either sex but especially the female when it may be recurrent with bouts of severe loin pain, tenderness, a high temperature and a variety of urinary symptoms. It is common in pregnancy, usually caused by a bacterial infection, either blood-transmitted or ascending via the ureters from an infected bladder (cystitis). The illness must be thoroughly diagnosed and treated to avoid a chronic condition with risks of renal impairment and circulatory complications.

REMEDIES

Aconitum, Berberis, Cantharis, Causticum, Hepar sulph., Mercurius, Sycotic Co.

Nervous illness

The commonest problem seen in our stress-laden society. It is present at all ages in all countries and involves every ethnic group. Nervousness reflects underlying emotional tension, stress, lack of confidence, uncertainty and fear. It is seen from childhood to old age and feeds on natural fears, uncertainties and anxieties concerned with war, social tensions and lack of physical or spiritual health and faith. Much of our present emotional stress is related to social and psychological pressures to be different, often trying to live up to an unreal media-ideal, or due to changes in the speed and rhythm of life. Many are ill-prepared for such pressures and quite unable to adapt or adjust, often from lack of training and education as to the best attitude and approach to take. Indeed there is no formal attention or education given, the emphasis on success in examinations rather than the broader needs of the individual and problem-solving in life as well as in the classroom. Flexibility, alternative solutions, adjustment to life's changes and problems are largely ignored and denied within our educational system to the personal loss of the individual. Homoeopathy can help enormously in some areas, supporting the underlying psychology. In all cases, a natural rhythm and overall mature approach to change and challenge is essential and must be fostered and supported throughout life.

REMEDIES

Arsenicum, Gelsemium, Ignatia, Lycopodium, Natrum mur., Nux vomica, Sulphur,

Neuralgia

This is a condition of local nerve pain often caused by an underlying physical problem, such as dental neuralgia. The cause is not always apparent. There is irritation of nerves in the affected area, often due to stress or a mechanical factors, e.g. an abscess or infection, shingles or arthritis, exposure to a draught. REMEDIES
Chamomilla, Coffea, Kalmia, Nux vomica, Rhus tox., Spigelia, Sulphur.

Neurosis

The common psychological condition where nervous symptoms due to stress intrude into everyday life and undermine relationships. Efficiency, concentration, joy, peace of mind - either at work or in home-relationships are absent, limited or sporadic. Common symptoms are physical ones, with recurrent colds, pains, chronic backache or fatigue. More obvious psychological symptoms are depression, hysteria, tearfulness, collapse, nausea and exhaustion. Phobias or obsessions may occur but not invariably. Often there is an inability to either build or sustain personal relationships, with loneliness, self-imposed isolation and a sense of guilt or futility. The underlying causes need to be explored, understood, verbalised, discussed and shared. There is no magic - and distorted assumptions or viewpoints about the motivations of others need to be replaced by more giving, interest, sharing and caring. In chronic problems, self-interest and self-protection has become more important than relationships and others.

REMEDIES
These include the specific constitutional prescription. For specifics, see section - Nervous illness.

Nitric Acid (Aqua fortis)

Indicated for an anxious, often depressed, thin, dark-complexioned person with skin problems especially around the junction-areas of skin and mucous membrane, as at the corners of the mouth or the ears or anal area. Typical symptoms are a fissure or fistula with sharp, cutting, stitch-like pains and a tendency to haemorrhage from an exposed fissure or ulcer. These areas are extremely tender and common inside the mouth and on the tongue as ulcers, usually worse for acid fruits and certain wines. Also for pneumonia, bronchitis, diarrhoea with blood in the stools as in typhus fever. There is severe pain on opening the bowels and attempting to pass a motion. The urine has a characteristic horse-like odour.

Nosode

Nosodes are prepared from diseased pathological tissue and used to prevent or treat a specific illness. First introduced by Lux (see section) in the face of much controversy, they are often of enormous value in treatment and without risk to the patient. They are of particular use in chronic conditions. A nosode should not usually be repeated for 6 months after the initial prescription. Examples include *Morbillinum,* (measles) *Varicellinum* (chicken-pox), *Tuberculinum bov* (Tuberculosis), *Anthracinum,* (Anthrax), *Medorrhinum* (gonorrhoea), *Pertussin* (whooping cough), the bowel nosodes of Bach and Paterson.

O

Obesity

The disease of excess weight seen in all ages but particularly prevalent in the middle years and 40 year age group. It is often associated with hormonal or psychological imbalance at a time when very profound physiological changes are occurring, with the extra stress of the 'mid-life' depressive crisis. Over the years, a pattern has usually developed of denying a particular problem area, by indulging in comfort eating in order to become calm in the face of the unknown. Food is reassuring and familiar, especially something sweet. The commonest reassurance-mechanism is undoubtedly food and creature comfort. Constantly repeating this reassuring comforting experience of eating throughout the day, together with lack of exercise, quickly contributes to body weight and size, often adding to depression. Organic causes include diabetes, Addison's disease, thyroid disorders especially Myxoedema and the side-effects of steroid drugs. Cardiac or renal failure with water retention are rarer contributory causes. Remedies must at all times take into account the underlying causes as well as the overall psychological and physical picture.
REMEDIES
Apis, Calcarea, Crataegus, Hamamelis, Kali carb., Phytolacca Berry, Thyroidinum.

Obsessional Neurosis

The psychological disorder where the major emphasis is control of 'self' and 'others' by rigid infantile magical thinking, psychological dogma and ritual. The aim of the obsessional defence, extensively described by Freud, is to prevent the buffeting and vicissitudes of life imposing upon the obsessional, catching him unawares, 'off-guard', so that he feels unprepared and in danger of being shown-up as a failure. Pride is strong and failure a terrifying nightmare. There is a multitude of fears and threats in every area of life. The rituals of avoiding cracks in the pavement, ladders, checking doors and gas taps is symbolic, to prevent being caught-out with his 'pants down'. This gives a clue to the infantile nature of its origins and the terror of being found defenceless and in a state of panic.

REMEDIES

Argentum nit., Gelsemium, Lycopodium, Natrum mur., Platina.

Ocimum Canum (Alfavaca)

Introduced to homoeopathy by Mure. It is a major remedy for right-sided renal colic where there is a red sandy deposit in the urine. Also for vomiting and collapse from renal colic, kidney stones, cystitis with infection, restlessness. The urine has a musk odour.

Oedema

Excess of fluid in the tissues of any part of the body, including the heart (pericardial oedema), lungs (pulmonary oedema), abdominal cavity (peritoneal oedema), limbs (ankle oedema), throat or soft palate (angioneurotic oedema). The most frequent type is oedema of the lower limb with ankle swelling, pitting on pressure, with swelling of the feet, ankles and legs. Symptoms are better for rest and in the mornings, worse for standing or fatigue. The legs feel heavy, like lead,

with pain, discomfort and slowness because of fluid retention. With the possible exception of lower limb oedema, all forms need treatment, often in hospital, by a physician. Leg oedema may be caused by many factors including:- cardiac weakness, heart failure, or kidney disease but most commonly a poor circulation from varicose veins. Other causes of leg swelling with oedema are:- phlebitis, local trauma, blockage of the lymphatic circulation, allergy and infection. Careful diagnosis and a detailed history is essential to exclude an obstructive condition which needs early referral for treatment. If there is a mechanical condition causing blockage, this must be dealt with by surgical correction, because any obstructive interference to flow and drainage, cannot usually be relieved by homoeopathy.
REMEDIES
Alumina, Apis, Calcarea, Hamamelis, Natrum mur., Pulsatilla, Sulphur.

Oestradiol (Prepared from the synthetic hormone)

This preparation is an effective treatment for many female menstrual problems. It is usually given daily in the 12x or 6c potency.

Oestrogen (The extract of the hormone)

This remedy is used increasingly for the effective alleviation of menopausal problems, e.g. hot flushes and as a homoeopathic substitute for hormone replacement therapy (H.R.T.). It is usually given daily throughout the female cycle, except during the time of menstrual bleeding.

Oleander (Rose Laurel)

Tincture of the leaves, first proved by Hahnemann. There is anxiety with faintness. Primarily this is a cardiac remedy with problems of severe palpitations, weakness, collapse and dizziness. Vertigo, diarrhoea, gastro-enteritis, are other common symptoms. The skin is raw, with rough chapping and soreness. Depression is the major emotional mood.

Onosmodium (False Gromwell)

Tincture of the fresh plant, first proved by Green in 1887. There is tension with irritability, the person impatient, in a hurry unable to relax as time passes so very slowly *(Medorrhinum)*. Both judgement and concentration are poor with accident proneness (Compare *Kali carb)*. Also for:- muscular weakness, inco-ordination, long-sightedness of the elderly, blurred double vision, eye strain, headaches, vertigo.

Operations - the use of homoeopathy in surgical procedures

It is advisable to take *Arnica* 30c both before and after an operation in order to reduce shock, swelling and bruising and to cut down the risk of haemorrhage. Arnica also helps to shorten the period of convalescent recovery. Usually one dose pre-operatively and two doses afterwards is sufficient. After major surgery, involving a large incision and post-operative pain, use *Staphysagria* after having first taken *Arnica*. For pre-operative fear and anxiety use *Argentum nit.* 30c three times daily during the 48 hour period preceding the operation. For post- operative chest conditions with a dry cough, pain and an irritating need to clear the throat constantly, give *Bryonia* three times daily until symptoms have been relieved. If a local inflammation develops post-operatively, e.g. with tender burning red streaks along an arm or limb, use *Belladonna* 6c three times daily, but also consult your doctor. In all cases the correct homoeopathic prescription makes the patient more comfortable and speeds recovery time.

Opium (Papaver Somniferum)

Tincture of the unripe poppy capsule. The main indications and symptoms are:- an acute cerebral catastrophe or 'stroke', with loss of consciousness, coma, pin-point fixed pupils and immobility. The face is bloated with a purple cyanotic hue and there may be vomiting, the breathing slow, laboured and noisy. Also for:- drowsiness, confusion, falling-about with unsteadiness or delirium. Constipation is total, with flatus passed. There is a lack of reaction in all areas, including to pain. It is also indicated for snoring.

Orchitis

Inflammation of the testicle. Commonly associated with infection by the mumps virus, either in childhood or the adult. The latter causes a more severe reaction and illness, sometimes leading to sterility. In some cases the origin is unknown and due to trauma or other infective agents. There is typically pain, swelling and discomfort.
REMEDIES
Clematis, Hamamelis, Pulsatilla, Rhododendron, Spongia.

Organic Illness

As opposed to emotional or psychological illness, there is pathology or disease in an organ or part of the body creating interference with normal functioning and leading to blockage and interference with the physiology of the part affected. The illness may also affect the central nervous system and cause interference with the normal psychological state, or the symptoms themselves provoke reactions of fear and anxiety because they are unfamiliar, not understood or seem illogical. An organic illness may not be amenable to homoeopathic treatment, depending upon the degree of obstruction and interference with normal functioning. A cyst or goitre may put pressure on surrounding tissues or underlying passageways, i.e. the oesophagus causing problems of swallowing in addition to interference with thyroid functioning. Surgery is required to relieve the obstruction, whatever homoeopathic treatment is given. Homoeopathy works well in organic illness provided the remedy is correctly prescribed according to overall symptoms. There is often correction of underlying disease in the area affected provided that it is not chronic or obstructive and sufficient vital energy is present. As with all illness, an overall total evaluation of the patient, symptoms and pathology must be considered. A surgical opinion is advisable in all cases, especially where severe scarring or obstruction undermines the ability of the homoeopathic remedy to function fully.

Organon - of Hahnemann

The Organon of the Rational System of Medicine - the title taken from Aristotle as the instrument of all reasoning. First published in Leipzig in 1810, it is the most important book published by Hahnemann. It sets out the whole of his philosophy of homoeopathy and its rules of application to the patient, laws of similitude and cure. The book was well received by homoeopaths the world over and has become a classic. There are six known editions, of which the last edition is the most important because of the footnotes and appendices. The *Organon* deserves a place on the bookshelf of every serious student of homoeopathy.

Ornithogalum Umbellatum (Star of Bethlehem)

Tincture of the fresh plant. Indicated for:- chronic digestive problems, burning pain with distention, flatulence and peptic ulceration. Especially the upper abdominal area is distended a short time after eating the smallest meal. Vomiting and heartburn are common. The predominant mood is depression and irritability

Ortega, Proceso S. M. D.

The eminent contemporary Mexican homoeopath and teacher. Founder of the Mexican teaching academy for the expansion of homoeopathy - *Homoeopatia de Dedico,* he has been an active teacher and physician within the International League for the past 20 years. Also director of the Mexican Journal *La Homoeopatia en el Mundo*, Vice-president of the International League. In two international congresses, (1981/82) his group has presented papers on the chronic miasms.

Osteoporosis

Decalcification or thinning of bone with increased liability to fractures. It is a common condition of the elderly. The bones on X-ray are almost transparent from loss of calcium. It also occurs after drug abuse, or indiscriminate vitamin therapy, over a prolonged period.
REMEDIES
Baryta carb., Calcarea Phos., Natrum mur., Symphytum.

Otitis Media

Acute inflammation of the middle ear, with severe pain, discharge of pus or mucus, especially when the drum has burst from internal pressure on the membrane. The temperature is high, the patient restless, at times toxic. It can be a most distressing recurrent childhood illness.
REMEDIES
Belladonna, Ferrum phos., Hepar sulph., Mercurius, Pulsatilla, Sulphur.

Ovarian Problems

For ovarian cyst, consider *Apis* when the cyst is right-sided with burning, stinging pains. *Lachesis* is more indicated for left-sided cyst and pains. For ovarian pain, unrelated to cystic conditions, but more to inflammation and hormonal disfunction use *Apis* or *Belladonna.* For pain at ovulation, consider *Colocynth, Naja, or Sabina.*

Oxalic Acid (Sorrel Acid)

Indicated for painful conditions particularly of the rheumatoid type. Most symptoms are left-sided but can occur in any part of the body. There are agonizing, sharp, severe pains worse from thinking or worrying about the condition. Exhaustion, weakness and collapse with coldness and shock is characteristic. Vomiting of blood may occur and there is a general bleeding tendency with small red spots or petechiae from minute haemorrhages under the skin. In some cases the condition proceeds to one of excitation or fits, but usually exhaustion and prostration dominate the picture.

P

Paeonia (Peony)

Tincture of the fresh root. This is a remedy for circulatory irregularities, with profuse hot-flushes, sweats, blushing of face, trunk and head. The anus is a problem area with splinter-like pains from anal fissure, fistula or haemorrhoids. Bed sores, itching and irritation is marked and all symptoms are worse for movement of any kind. The major mental symptoms are severe restlessness or fearfulness with nightmares. All symptoms are better for rest and aggravated by walking or movement.

Pain

Perhaps the most distressing of all human suffering. It varies very considerably both in degree and character, also frequency, site, time of onset, aggravating factors, duration and causation.

REMEDIES

Aconite severe acute pain with restlessness and marked fear.

Arnica the pain has a bruised-like quality.

Arsenicum pain is acute and burning with severe agitation.

Belladonna the pain red-hot, worse for touch but better for local pressure on the affected part.

Bryonia the pain worse for the least movement or jarring.

Cactus for vice-like and cramping pains.

Colocynth for severe colicky pain, better for doubling-up.

Glonoin pain is throbbing and beating.

Nitric acid pains are splinter-like, sharp or burning.
Nux vom. pain is sporadic, cramping with anger and marked irritability.
Rhus tox. pain is relieved by heat and movement.
Staphysagria the pain is sharp, tearing, often post-operational with a marked feeling of resentment.

Palpitations

Heightened awareness of the heart's action, usually with increased rapidity or irregularity of the heart-beat. Shock or emotional pressure and stress are common causes of palpitations. Symptoms come on during the day or night, often at rest. There may be additional psychological tension because of fear of heart disease. Excesses of tea or coffee throughout the day often provoke a similar quickening of the heart rate. Other causes are:- viral infection, degeneration or blockage of the conducting pathways and various metabolic diseases, including an over-active thyroid.
REMEDIES
Crataegus, Naja, Nux vomica, Spigelia.

Pancreatitis

Acute inflammation of the pancreas, usually from infective causes. Symptoms are of the most severe abdominal pain, cramping and unbearable, with collapse and shock. Most cases need urgent hospitalisation and sometimes surgery.
REMEDIES
Aconitum, Atropine, Iodum, Iris, Kali hydriod.

Paracelsus (1490 - 1541)

The philosopher and forerunner of Hahnemann who found a specific relationship between certain plant and mineral remedies and symptoms of disease. He described the Simillimum principle and advocated treatment of 'like by like'. He was able to effect impressive cures by these principles and is regarded as an innovator, a man far in advance of his time.

Paralysis

The illness may be acute and sudden, as from a 'stroke' due to a cerebral thrombosis, raised blood-pressure or a haemorrhage. Also infection, e.g. poliomyelitis, arteriosclerosis, trauma - as when a nerve is severed. Variable weakness or paralysis occurs in multiple sclerosis. Other causes include degenerative disease - sometimes hereditary or of unknown causation like Motor Neurone Disease.

REMEDIES

Arnica for shock.

Opium for stroke paralysis and unconsciousness.

Natrum mur. for Multiple Sclerosis.

Paris for left-sided paralysis.

Phosphorus for degenerative condition.

Spartium for raised blood-pressure.

Veratrum alb. for severe collapse with shock and pallor.

Pareira (Virgin Vine)

Tincture of the fresh root, first proved by Fox. The main site of action is the urinary tract, with severe cystitis, urgency, burning pains, strangury (pain at the end of the passage of water), also for urinary retention, urethritis and dysuria (pain on passing water). Prostate problems are a further indication to prescribe.

Paris Quadrifolia (One Berry)

Tincture of the whole fruiting plant, first proved by Hahnemann. It acts on mucous membrane, especially of the eyes, helping conjunctivitis with pain and a sensation of the eyeballs protruding as in thyroid disease. There is an offensive diarrhoea. It is mainly a left-sided remedy, the mind irritable, overactive and talkative *(Compare Lachesis).*

Parkinsonism (Paralysis Agitans)

The chronic, degenerative nervous condition, usually of the elderly, with fine tremor, pill-rolling movements of thumbs and an associated increase of joint-stiffness and resistance to movement. The body is slow in motion, functioning and speech with thinking and responses generally retarded. Response to homoeopathy is often slow or limited where there is severe degeneration of major conducting pathways.
REMEDIES
Arsenicum, Baryta carb., Nux vomica, Phosphorus, Zinc. met.

Parotidinum (The mumps nosode)

The remedy made from infected parotid glandular tissue and often used prophylactically. It is of especial value when there are vulnerable adults in contact with the disease, who have not been previously affected and therefore have no immunity. The illness is mainly severe in the adult and it can be used to advantage in the 30c potency when there are complications, as a high temperature, orchitis, mastitis or meningitis.

Paschero, Tomas Pablo. M.D. (1904 -)

The eminent Buenos Aires homoeopath and co-founder of the Argentinean Homoeopathic Medical Association since 1934. An authority on the importance of *The Organon* in Homoeopathic literature as also, the role of psychological factors and the mentals in homoeopathy. He has contributed many important papers in this field at International Congresses. *The Mental Symptoms in Homoeopathy* (1975) is of especial importance.

Passiflora Incarnata (Passion flower)

Introduced by Hale (see section) to homoeopathy. It is a useful remedy for spasmodic conditions with violent contractions. Also for:- tetanus, epilepsy, puerperal convulsions, asthma, whooping cough, manic states of excitement and delirium tremens.

Paterson, Elizabeth. M.D. (1907-1963)

Wife and co-worker of John Paterson, who did so much to establish the importance of the bowel nosodes in prescribing. A Glasgow graduate, she practised homoeopathy with her husband and they spent most of their lives working and teaching in Glasgow. Working with Dishington and Wheeler (see section), influenced by Bach, they formed the key workers who separated the major characteristics of *Morgan, Gaertner, and Sycotic Co.*

Major writings include:
1935 Chronic miasms and prescribing
1941 Nutrition
1959 A Survey of the Nosodes

Paterson, John. M.D. (1890-1954)

The eminent Glasgow homoeopathic teacher and researcher. President of the International League and President of the Homoeopathic faculty. His general papers include - *Hahnemann's doctrine of Psora, The Homoeopathic treatment of skin diseases.* He followed Dishington as physician at the Glasgow children's hospital Mount Vernon and continued his pioneering work. Together with his wife Elizabeth, they established the clinical indications for such important bowel nosodes as *Dysentery Co, Morgan, Gaertner, and Sycotic Co.* This entirely new group of remedies, developed from the non-lactose fermenting bacteria, normally present in the bowel, are of enormous clinical importance and have widely extended the range and scope of the homoeopathic pharmacy.

Pertussin (Coqueluchin)

The nosode of the whooping cough virus, used very effectively in the prevention and treatment of the disease without the risks of conventional vaccine treatment to the nervous system. It is often given from the 6th month onwards.

Petroleum (Coal Oil)

Trituration of rectified oil. First proved by Hahnemann (see section), it is a major anti-psora remedy, indicated for skin symptoms where there is chronic eczema with soreness and redness with itching. Deep red cracks are common. The mood is one of peevish irritability, flaring-up into outbursts of anger and rage. Nausea and headaches in the occiput (posterior head area) are characteristic, all symptoms aggravated by cold or movement.

Petroselinum (Parsley)

Tincture of the fresh plant. First proved by Bethmann it acts mainly on the urinary system for problems of:- cystitis, bladder irritability, urgency and burning pain on passing water. It also acts on gonorrhoeal urethritis with a creamy or yellow discharge and prostatic enlargement with frequency.

Petzinger, Von Karl Johann. M.D.

The eminent German physician and homoeopath, who worked mainly in Konigsberg. Past chairman of the regional association of homoeopathic doctors of Nieder-Sachsen and from 1959, chairman of the self-dispensing homoeopathic doctors. He was active in the International League as a teacher and organiser for many years.

Pharyngitis

Inflammation of the pharynx or soft tissues at the back of the throat and mouth, usually infective in origin. The condition may be either acute or chronic. Major symptoms are pain on swallowing, general soreness and redness of the area, with an infected yellowish-green mucus dripping into the back of the throat. The area feels hot and swollen. There is often a high temperature, the lymph nodes, enlarged and tender.

REMEDIES

For acute cases consider:- *Aconitum, Belladonna, Lachesis, Mercurius, Phytolacca.*

For chronic cases consider:- *Argentum nit., Baryta carb., Sulphur.*

Phelan, Richard. M.D. (1836 - 1902)

The Irish-born homoeopathic physician who treated Kent's (see section) wife in St Louis and later became his tutor. He founded the Hering Medical College of St Louis in 1880, which later merged with the homoeopathic Medical College St Louis.

Phellandrium (Water drop wort)

The major spheres of action is on the breast and respiratory tissues. Mainly a right-sided remedy, it is indicated in chronic bronchitis and emphysema, with chronic cough and shortness of breath. Mucus production is often offensive and infected. Headache is common and the head feels too large. Pain in the nipples between feeds when lactating, is characteristic.

Phlebitis

Inflammation of the veins. The condition should always be treated medically because of the danger of embolus formation. The condition may be superficial, from a local wound or bite, or sometimes there is a more generalised infection with involvement of the deep veins. The latter condition needs careful attention and medical care. In some cases anticoagulant therapy is required. The condition of deep vein thrombosis may follow any operation or a severe prolonged physical illness with lengthy period of bed-rest. Symptoms are:- shooting pains in the area, a raised temperature with swelling, redness, tenderness or stiffness.
REMEDIES
Aconitum, Hamamelis, Lachesis, Phosphorus, Pulsatilla, Vipera.

Phleum Pratense (Timothy grass)

For hay-fever due to sensitivity to grass pollens, associated with tightness of the chest or asthma. It can be used as a prophylactic in early cases. The classic symptoms occur each year, usually in the late spring or early summer, with sneezing, a watery nasal discharge and itchy irritation of the nose and eyes.

Phosphoric Acidum (Phosphoric acid)

First proved by Hahnemann. The remedy has marked action on the emotions, in particular symptoms of fatigue, exhaustion, drowsiness with depression. In contrast to *Opium,* the patient is more easily roused from a stupor-like state of apathy. Most of the excretory areas of the body are stimulated to drain and discharge profusely and there is a frequent passage of urine. It is of value for the morose, grief-stricken or depressed, when unable to rally or respond to reassurance and support (Compare *Ignatia)*.

Phosphorus (White phosphorus)

The remedy for sudden violent explosive outbursts of symptoms with burning pains. It is indicated for:- tall, pale, fair or red-haired constitutions, often thin and anaemic-looking. There are many chest symptoms, with cough, bronchitis, asthma, pneumonia, shortness of breath, blood in the sputum and flashes of burning pains in the stomach or intestine. Also for diarrhoea and vomiting of mucus. They crave salt and ice-cold drinks.

Physostigma (Calabar Bean)

A remedy for spasm as in tetanus, spinal paralysis, poliomyelitis and spinal meningitis. Also for vomiting, collapse, diarrhoea with a slow pulse, palpitations and sweating. The pupil is pin-point as after a stroke. Useful in any chronic paralysing conditions such as:- multiple sclerosis, motor neurone disease, hereditary ataxias with weakness, muscle wasting, loss of strength and power.

Phytolacca Decandra (Poke Root)

Tincture of the fresh root, first introduced to homoeopathy by Hale (see section) and one of the best remedies for:- violent throat pain with soreness and swelling of the soft palate and pharynx. Other indications are:- pain on swallowing and tonsillitis, diphtheria, vomiting and diarrhoea, muscular cramps, rigidity, spasm or convulsions. The other main sphere of action is breast tissue i.e. mastitis, cystic nodular breast problems, or a cracked nipple with soreness. The breasts are usually painful during the menstrual periods.

Pilocarpinum (Jaborandi)

An alkaloid, which in homoeopathic form is indicated for mumps, night-sweats of the menopause and in overactive thyroid disease (hyperthyroidism). Restless irritability is common. The remedy is recommended for many eye problems, especially fatigue, a contracted pupil, lachrymation (irritation), short-sightedness.

Placebo

An inert, non-medicated substance (lactose or sucrose), which is sometimes prescribed to observe the patient for a period without medication or to allow a prescribed remedy a greater period of prolonged action, without interference. It is often used where it is felt that the patient, during the interim waiting stage, needs psychological support. According to how the physician best judges the psychological needs and strengths of the patient, a placebo may or may not be required.

Plantago (Plantain)

Tincture of the whole fresh plant. Introduced by Hale to homoeopathy. It is a rather unusual remedy in that it is often used locally as the undiluted mother-tincture for toothache or painful haemorrhoids. Of especial value in abscess, dental neuralgia, trigeminal (cranial nerve) neuralgia and for earache. It is also indicated where large amounts of urine are passed, as in diabetes or enuresis. It relieves the severe pain of piles when they are inflamed. It is a left-sided remedy, all symptoms worse from cold air, movement, or excessive heat.

Platina (the metal Platinum)

Trituration of the element. Platina is a major remedy for hysteria and pride associated with depression, irritability and restlessness. There may be impulses to violence. Cramps, spasm, constipation and pruritis vulvae, are other symptoms which suggest the remedy.

Plumbum Met (Lead)

Trituration of the element. It is an important remedy which acts on paralysis of certain groups of muscles, especially with wrist-drop or weakness. Pains are severe, cramping or wandering, with spasm of a colicky type. Constipation is absolute. Also for anal spasm and gout. The patient is emaciated with loss of weight and exhaustion. There is a characteristic greyish-blue tinge to the skin. All symptoms are better from rest, warmth and firm local pressure. The typical lead colic is improved by local heat to the area and for doubling-up.

Pneumonia

Inflammation of the lung by either bacterial or viral infection. This is a serious condition with a raised temperature, except in the elderly when it may be below normal. Symptoms include:- a painful cough, blood in the sputum, shortness of breath, weakness or collapse. It is best treated by a physician or hospitalisation.
REMEDIES
Aconitum, Arsenicum, Lycopodium, Mercurius, Rhus tox., Senega, Sulphur.

Podophyllum (May-apple)

Tincture of the whole plant, first proved by Williamson. There are many bowel symptoms with griping, colicky abdominal pain, flatulence, weakness and diarrhoea. The stools are watery or greenish and after their passage the patient feels faint. Also for:- rectal or uterine prolapse, right-sided ovarian pain, vomiting of pregnancy and haemorrhoids of pregnancy.

Poisoning

Acute poisoning may be accidental or deliberately induced. The commonest causes are:- infected or contaminated food as mushroom poisoning, botulism from infected tinned food. Food poisoning is usually caused by a *salmonella* organism. Carbon monoxide from fumes and engine exhaust gases, causes asthma and bronchitis. It is a common problem in busy inner urban areas. In poorly ventilated areas, domestic gas may be a toxic hazard, and gas fires should be checked regularly as every year fatalities occur. Other forms of poisoning are the ingestion of toxic chemical substances used in the home. It is particularly dangerous to store weed killer or caustic fluids in a lemonade or beer bottle. Sedatives taken to excess cause toxic confusion and illness. Alcohol poisoning may occur when large quantities of strong alcohol are consumed rapidly - either in error or for bravado. The acute cases must be treated urgently, under medical care. Depending upon the cause, vomiting should be induced by means of an emetic made from salt, or mustard and water. The patient must be removed from the toxic area and treated for shock and kept warm.

Chronic poisoning is often due to atmospheric pollution, causing urban asthma in children. Other environmental hazards are:- nitrates and lead, often at dangerous unacceptable levels, D.D.T., now globally distributed, radioactive cobalt and strontium, now found in the foetus and newborn child. Symptoms must be treated by the most appropriate remedy, such as political lobbying, and the avoidance of densely populated urban areas whenever possible.

REMEDIES

Aconitum, Arnica, Rescue Remedy, Veratrum alb.

Poliomyelitis (Infantile paralysis)

The acute viral illness with infiltration and inflammation of the spinal cord nerve roots leading to degeneration, paralysis and wasting of certain muscle groups according to the degree of spinal root infiltration. Depending upon the severity of the attack, the disease may affect facial, laryngeal, respiratory or limb muscles with weakness, wasting, or complete paralysis. It is highly infective and still endemic in some third world countries, but preventable by the specific poliomyelitis vaccine. In recent years the disease has become rare in Europe although still a risk in some areas. In all cases medical care is needed and hospitalisation when severe.

REMEDIES *Arsenicum, Baryta carb, Calcarea carb., Gelsemium, Phosphorus.*

Pollen Sensitivity

Often an inherited problem with a family history of hay-fever, asthma or eczema in one or both parents. The person affected is usually of a sensitive nature, both psychologically and physiologically. Stress or anxiety heightens physical discomfort. The commonest problems are:- hay fever with conjunctivitis, itchy red eyes, itchy palate, sneezing, nasal congestion and tightness of the chest with asthma. In some cases the condition may become unrelated to pollen and more linked to dust, animal hair, or hot dry conditions, sometimes present all the year around.
REMEDIES
Dulcamara, House dust, Kali carb., Phleum pratense, Mixed pollens, Phosphorus.

Polyps

Enlargement and prolongation of the mucosa can occur in any part of the body where there is a mucous membrane lining, including the large bowel, uterus, bladder and nasal mucosa. It is a frequent cause of bleeding and discharge with irritation and blockage in the area. The commonest area affected is the nose with swelling and oedema, chronic nasal catarrh, mouth breathing, epistaxis (nose bleeding) and infective discharges. The polyps can frequently be seen on examination of the nostril.
REMEDIES
Calc. carb., Kali bich., Mercurius, Phosphorus, Sanguinaria, Thuja.

Porter, Eugene. M.D. (1856 - 1929)

The 19th century homoeopath who graduated from the New York Homoeopathic Medical College in 1885, where he became Professor of Materia Medica (1902). He was editor of The North American Journal of Homoeopathy (1892-1897).

Potency - homoeopathic

Refers to the strength or dilution of the remedy at each stage of its preparation. The higher the potency - for example a 200c or 10^{-400} dilution - the stronger the remedy. Each successive dilution, dynamised by the succussion process, enhances the strength, activity, depth and breadth of action of the remedy. The polycrests and constitutional remedies are commonly prescribed in the higher 200c potencies, whilst a remedy used for a more local condition is given in the lower 6c dilution. Potency is the innate energy-factor used in the medicines - ultimately one of natures deepest and most effective catalyst-elements. A recent paper at the international congress of Vienna, emphasised just these points. Gutman and Resch were able to demonstrate that homoeopathic potency is something quite different from the usual physical principles and models used, which are largely experimental, but do not occur as such in nature or man. Potency is not measurable by conventional instruments designed to pick up energy charges of a different type. During trituration and succussion, a dynamic pattern is liberated which the solvent memorises, affecting molecular energy and giving a far greater speed of movement. This memory can be transmitted to glass, as has been known to the homoeopathic pharmacist for many years. It is present when water is used as a diluent, but enhanced by an alcohol mixture and succussion. Gutman and Resch recommended the centesimal scale of dilution as being more effective than the decimal scale in the transmission of potency energy charges.

Pregnancy

There are no contra-indications to the use of homoeopathic remedies during pregnancy and it can be quite safely prescribed for morning sickness (*Cocculus, Nux Vom.*), miscarriage and threatened abortion of the 3rd month *(Caulophyllum, Sabina, Secale, Sepia).* Problems of the pregnant mother based on anxiety or fear, tension, apprehension or intercurrent physical illness, can also be treated without risk to mother or baby. In the last four months of the pregnancy, *Caulophyllum* is given to stimulate healthy uterine tone and functioning, to make for a healthy smooth labour and delivery.

Prevention by homoeopathy

It is well-recognized that homoeopathy has an important role to play in prevention. The chances of contacting a specific infection from a child or neighbour, may need to be minimised for a variety of reasons. Examples include:- *Belladonna* for measles prevention, *Pertussin* for whooping cough, *Mercurius cy.* for diphtheria. The nosodes of mumps, German measles, glandular fever, chicken-pox have a similar prophylactic action.

Primula veris (Cowslip)

Tincture of the fresh whole plant. The remedy is of value for cerebral congestion, drowsiness or dullness with disorientation and confusion. Also for unsteadiness from a threatened 'stroke' or cerebral catastrophe, when the blood-pressure becomes high and critical. The head is hot and there is a headache with dizziness and a sensation of fullness.

Principles of Homoeopathy

The science of homoeopathy is based on two major principles which are basic to the method:
1. A comparative study is made of the manifestations or external symptoms of the illness, with those produced by the medical substances used in the treatment. This is called the Law of Similitudes when the two symptom patterns of patient and remedy are matched by the prescriber. For example, coffee in its homoeopathic form of *Coffea,* can be used in the treatment of insomnia, palpitations and agitation.
2. The therapeutic use of infinitesimal dosages, produced by successive serial dilutions of the mother tincture and free from any possible toxic side-effects of the medicaments used. Such substances are traditionally of vegetable, plant, animal or mineral origin.

Progesterone (Synthetic extract of the hormone)

This remedy is useful for female menstrual problems, helping to regularise problems of hormonal imbalance.

Prostate Problems

These include:- acute prostatitis from bacterial or viral infection with pain and tenderness in the area, urinary irritation and discomfort. The commonest difficulty is benign prostatic enlargement of middle-aged and elderly males causing delay, difficulty in passing urine, frequency and a weak stream. Careful examination is necessary in order to avoid missing the rarer malignant growth of prostate which may give similar symptoms.
REMEDIES
Chamomilla, Digitalis, Eupatorium purp., Ferrum pic., Mercurius, Sabal Serrulata, Solidago.

Proteus (Bach)

The bowel nosode for dark-haired, tense and irritable depressive temperaments prone to violent attacks of temper if crossed. Impulsive, sudden, with poor controls they are equally spasmodic in every area of functioning. There may be sudden spasms in the blood supply to an area, with angina, coronary thrombosis, intermittent claudication, capillary spasm with 'dead' fingers. Violent flashes of heat occur, also indigestion with a sour taste, acidity, heartburn and hunger pains are typical. Constipation is a common problem, also anal itching. It is recommended for tendon contractures *(Compare Causticum),* especially of the palms and little finger. Cramp, sudden and violent, with associated irritability, is a further indication for the remedy.

Provings

The experimental use of a homoeopathic potency by healthy volunteers, who carefully record the results of taking different strengths of substance, over a period of several weeks. Careful daily record is kept of all symptoms experienced including any sensitivity to the remedy, or a vigorous response. The totality is put together to complete the remedy picture and indications for prescribing. The first early provings were carried out by Hahnemann on his family and colleagues, the remedy known to the provers. In recent years to avoid suggestion playing a role, the tendency has been to carry out double-blind proving trials, where neither provers, nor the physician in charge, knows the identity of the remedy until after the experiment. With a totally new remedy of no known or published results, a double-blind proving is still necessary, to eliminate possible 'placebo' symptoms of the prover.

Pruritus

Itching of the skin, particularly common in the anal-genital area, although it can occur in any part of the body. It is a distressing common problem and may be associated with haemorrhoids, varicose veins, allergy, or infection. Threadworm is common in adults as well as children, the itching characteristically occurring at night. A period of prolonged stress and strain may cause pressure and emotional tension, which finds relief and a temporary outlet, by scratching at an area of intolerable itching.
REMEDIES
Caladium, Cina, Hamamelis, Rhus tox., Rumex crisp.

Psora

The most important of Hahnemann's three hereditary miasms, extensively developed in detail in his writings on *Chronic Disease.* It is considered that Psora developed in a major way, as a result of suppression of the 'itch' or scabies infection and according to Hahnemann this is the root of many of our present chronic disease problems. Major symptoms involve the skin with infection, cracking, also diarrhoea and chronic indigestion is common. Depression, apathy with exhaustion are other manifestations of psora.
REMEDIES
Arsenicum, Aurum, Baryta carb., Calcarea carb., Carbo veg., Causticum, Graphites, Hepar sulph., Kali carb., Mezereum, Petroleum, Phosphorus, Sulphur, Psorinum.

Psoriasis

The now common skin condition of unknown origin, occurring in all age groups from childhood onwards. There are multiple areas of eruption with isolated thickened red patches which join-up, and may cover the entire body or an old area of injury. They have a silvery covering layer which tends to flake easily, causing itching and general discomfort. The lesions are disfiguring, but usually completely heal without scar formation. During the acute phase, the face, scalp, trunk or limbs may be involved and cause psychological problems because of their unsightly nature. The nails, hands, joints or genital area, are also often involved.
REMEDIES
Calcarea, Graphites, Kali arsen., Mezereum. Natrum mur., Petroleum, Psorinum, Pulsatilla.

Psorinum (Scabies)

The nosode of psora, prepared from the infected scabies vesicle. It is one of the most valuable of all remedies. The main indications are:- lack of concentration, depression with despair, an infected 'itch' which discharges, or chronic skin conditions, with offensive oozing and infection. There is general chilliness, the skin dirty-looking, sweat offensive and also the diarrhoea. Insatiable canine hunger is characteristic, plus weakness and shortness of breath on exertion.

Ptelea Trifoliata (Water Ash)

A useful remedy for hepatitis and chronic liver problems, where there is tenderness and enlargement. The liver area feels painful, like a dragging weight, pulling down the whole of the right upper abdominal region. The person feels uncomfortable and worse for lying on the right side. Also for chronic indigestion and rheumatic problems, usually right-sided (Compare *Lycopodium).*

Puberty

The onset of breast changes and the menstrual cycle in the girl, secondary sexual changes, pubic hair and emissions in the boy, as a preparation for reproduction and adult life. It is a time of major hormonal and psychological adjustment. The age of onset is getting younger in successive generations, as the general health and nutrition of the population improves. The average age of menstrual onset is now from 12-14 years with a wide range of difference on either side of this figure. When early periods are delayed, or variable and irregular, *Pulsatilla* is often of help. Where the child is late in developing generally and sexual development is retarded, consider *Calcarea carb.* or *Silicea.*

Pulsatilla Nigrans (Anemone Pratensis)

Tincture of the fresh flowering plant. The remedy is indicated whenever there is great change and variability of mood or symptoms, and is especially helpful in the female, although not solely. The temperament is passive, compliant, frequently tearful but at the same time quickly changing to stubbornness and anger before returning to becoming the peacemaker and usually being too easy-going. There are many digestive catarrhal problems with exhaustion, chilliness and discomfort on the warmest day. Profuse weeping is a common feature. Because of considerable congestion and a tendency to fluid retention, thirst is usually completely lacking. Fats are as disagreeable to *Pulsatilla* as heat and both, cause suffering and discomfort.

Q

Quin, Harvey Foster. M.D. (1799-1878)

The eminent homoeopath who first introduced homoeopathy to this country. He was particularly impressed by the approach at an early age, soon after qualifying and especially by the results of homoeopathy in the Paris cholera epidemic of 1831. He had enormous influence on our earliest English homoeopaths and formed the first English Homoeopathic Society in 1837. He was founder-president of the British Homoeopathic Society in 1844. The London Homoeopathic Hospital was also formed under his influence in 1844 where he began teaching and held comprehensive courses of clinical tuition.
Major writings include:
1838 Materia Medica Pura

Quinsy

The condition of peritonsillar abscess, usually on one side only, with a high temperature, severe pain, toxicity and a choking sensation. The tonsil area is severely inflamed and enlarged, the child ill, with vomiting and sometimes collapsing from fever. Fortunately the condition has now become rare.
REMEDIES
Aconitum, Baryta carb., Hepar sulph., Mer. sol., Silicea, Sulphur.

R

Rademacher, Johann Gottfried. M.D. (1772-1850)

The early medical practitioner, working mainly from Goch in North-Western Germany during the first half of the 19th century. He was a keen observer, disciple and admirer of Paracelsus. In 1841 he published his major work in German - *Universal and Organ Remedies* in two volumes, 800 pages each. Here he developed his principles and theory of organ correspondences, or remedies having special affinity for certain parts of the body. He was important because his ideas affected medical thinking for several generations and he firmly laid the emphasis of disease on the organ involved and the pathology of disease, also in chronic illness. To this extent he was in opposition to Hahnemann's ideas of more overall symptoms, including the mentals and modalities being of key importance for prescribing. Rademacher was supported by both Hughes, Burnett and others. See for example Burnett's monographs on *Diseases of the Liver and Spleen.*

Raeside, John Robertson. M.D. (1926-1972)

One of the victims of the tragic Trident air disaster of 1972 which took so many young and promising homoeopaths, travelling together to the Brussels International Congress of that year. Raeside especially was pre-eminent in his group. Born in Glasgow and educated in that city, he had a natural sensitivity towards the philosophy of Steiner, which he supported all his life. Formerly assistant to Dr. Blackie, he played an important role in the field of new remedy provings and gave a revival of interest to a difficult area, with a series of well-presented and scientific papers over several years. He was the spearhead of research at the Faculty up to the time of his death.

Ranunculus Bulb (Buttercup)

Essentially a remedy for muscular rheumatism with stitching, tearing pains of chest and spine. The symptoms are aggravated by fear (compare *Aconitum*). The patient feels weak and faint. Also for pleurisy, with burning pains on breathing-in, all symptoms aggravated by damp or cold air. The same burning pains may involve the bladder or stomach. The remedy is also helpful for chronic alcoholism with hiccup, shingles, skin irritation problems with redness, vesicle (blister) formations which are itchy and irritable.

Raphanus Sativus (the Black Radish)

Flatulence with a sensation of a bubble of air in the stomach that cannot be released (compare *Kali carb.*). It is specially valuable in post-operative paralysis or atony of the alimentary tract.

Ratanhia (Krameria)

Tincture of the root. The remedy acts on the large bowel with constipation and hard, dry, painful, stools causing straining and pressure and leading to severe haemorrhoids. The piles are painful and burning after a motion. There are two bizarre, but characteristic and diagnostic symptoms:- the rectum feels like splinters of glass (compare *Thuja)* and the back teeth have a sensation of cold water running through them.

Rau, Martin Gotleib. (1779- 1841)

The early German homoeopathic physician and author of *The Organon of Specific Homoeopathy.*

Raue, Charles Gottlieb. M.D. (1820-1896)

The early 19th century German homoeopathic physician who came to the US in 1850. He was a friend of Hering and co-editor of Hering's *Guiding Symptoms,* he wrote some of the earliest and most important volumes on psychology emphasising the importance of the mentals for prescribing.

Major writings include:

1868 Subjective and Objective symptoms

1868 Special Pathological and diagnosis

1870 Mental symptoms

1871 Elements of Psychology

1870-75 The annual record of homoeopathic literature

1884 A memorial of Constantine Hering

1889 Psychology as a natural science

Rauwolfia (Apocyanea)

A recently proved remedy for the treatment of irritable depression and raised blood-pressure, with palpitations. Also for headache and shortness of breath.

Raynaud's Disease

Arterial spasm from hypersensitivity of the circulatory system, usually due to cold. It occurs at any age, affecting particularly the hands, with the finger tips becoming lifeless and white. At other times the fingers are red, mauve, tingling and itching. The problem can occur in young men associated with excessive cigarette smoking. Often there is a family predisposition going back over several generations. Rarely, in the severe form of the disease, it can lead to gangrene and loss of limb.

REMEDIES

Agaricus, Nux vomica, Pulsatilla, Secale, Silicea.

Reactions to Homoeopathy

Deficient reactions, when there is only minimal improvement and only a short-lived response to the well-prescribed remedy may occur in the elderly with low vital energy levels. It sometimes occurs after a long illness which has depleted energy reserves from chronic illness, or where there is a mechanical and organic obstruction, with a surgical rather than a homoeopathic condition. For failure to respond, other than in obstructive problems, Boenninghausen (see section) recommended:- *Carbo veg., Laurocerasus, Opium, Sulphur, Thuja.* A nosode should also be considered e.g. *Medorrhinum, Psorinum, Tuberculinum Bov, Syphilinum.* Excessive reactions need a different approach. A severe aggravation sometimes occurs when steroids have been used - causing 'bounce-back' because symptoms have often been held down artificially and just under the surface, until the homoeopathic remedy comes into effect to release them. A 'Jack in the box' reaction occurs. Such excessive reactions are nearly always unavoidable and do not reflect wrong or inaccurate prescribing, but the start of a homoeopathic reaction. For severe initial reactions, after years of suppression, Boenninghausen recommended *Asafoetida, Chamomilla, China, Coffea, Ignatia, Nux Vom., Sulphur, Teucrium, Valerian.*

Reappearance of earlier Symptoms

During the course of homoeopathic treatment, it is quite common for earlier suppressed and usually inadequately treated illnesses, (sometimes from years previously), to re-emerge as isolated symptoms. Only rarely does it reappear as an illness, and it is usually transient and fragmentary in passage. Such symptoms are however important and significant, revealing that they have been underlying factors in the recent illness that has brought the patient for treatment. Once they have emerged and been treated by the appropriate homoeopathic prescription they tend not to recur. Examples are the recurrence of an old and forgotten gonorrhoeal infection which recurs as a discharge with no recent cause for it. Other symptoms seen are the return of hay-fever or transient asthma. The patient usually makes better progress once these underlying suppressed factors have come out and been dealt with.

Recovery by the Homoeopathic Method

Both patient and physician must fully realise that the response to homoeopathy follows a clear-cut order and natural law of response. In all cases, whatever the problem or remedy prescribed, recovery proceeds from the centre outwards. A cardiac symptom as angina, recovers before a joint or skin disability. It also occurs from above downwards, the scalp and face clearing in chronic psoriasis or eczema, before the trunk or limbs. Symptoms disappear in reverse order of appearance and the most recent are cured first, (those of longest duration last of all). It is not uncommon in heart disease for the patient to complain that he is no better. On close examination:- the palpitations, breathlessness and angina pain have quite gone, but the patient now has rheumatic pains. This means that the process of homoeopathic cure has begun exactly according to expectation, but the patient has quickly forgotten his earlier problems and now complains of being worse rather than better. He then risks being given another prescription for a condition that has really evolved and improved.

Rectal Prolapse

Protrusion of rectal mucosa, from lack of tone or muscular weakness may follow a debilitating illness, loss of weight, severe strain, surgery in the pelvic area, childbirth, or problems of chronic severe constipation.
REMEDIES
Argentum nit., Fluor. ac., Hydrastis, Phosphorus, Podophyllum, Syphilinum.

Renal Colic

The condition of severe abdominal pain due to the passage of a renal calculus along the ureter. The pain is cramping and unbearable, causing shock, weakness and collapse. The condition is usually eased by doubling-up and local heat.
REMEDIES
Berberis, Dioscorea, Magnesium phos., Nux vomica, Senecio, Urtica.

Repertory

The reference book of all homoeopathic physicians containing the totality of all the recorded proving symptoms, classified and related to the appropriate remedy and according to general and particular symptoms and their modalities. A patient is repertorised when the total symptom-picture is matched against the repertory listing, in order to decide which remedy fits the majority of the symptoms. The most extensive and best known repertories are those of Kent - which is widely used, and also that of Boenninghausen. In recent months the repertory has been computer-programmed for speed and convenience.

Repetition of the Remedy

It is a fundamental rule of homoeopathic practice not to repeat the prescribed remedy as long as the patient is improving. When prescribing for more local conditions in low 6c or 3x potencies, these should be stopped as soon as the condition has completely cleared. They should not be repeated again unless there is a recurrence of symptoms, when a different remedy is required.

Rescue Remedy (Bach)

This is a composite remedy, first made by Dr. Edward Bach to calm states of emotional emergency with tension and turmoil. It is made from the following wild flowers in alcohol solution: Impatiens (Impatiens glandulifera) for tension and stress, Clematis (Clematis vitalba) for vague disassociation states, Rock Rose (Helianthemum mummularium) for tension and pain, Cherry plum (Prunus cerasifera) for desperation, Star of Bethlehem (Ornithogalum umbellatum) for acute shock.

Resonance

The homoeopathic concept of the affinity of a specific remedy for the particular patient and his unique patterns of symptoms and needs at a given time. When the remedy is 'right' and matches the patient, it is in resonance and a vital reaction occurs, manifested by external changes in the symptom-pattern and an increase in available energy and well-being. At deeper levels, there is also a change in the internal dynamics, with a freeing of fixed areas of stress or non-functioning, beginning with the most recent, uppermost layers of rigidity and stasis. This freeing will always occur, provided that the problem is not of a mechanical nature that requires surgery.

Rest - importance of

During the course of homoeopathic treatment, regular habits are recommended with a rhythmic life and routine. Avoidance of excesses, including tea, coffee, tobacco and highly spiced foods is advisable and attention should be given to the quality and amount of food taken. This is to encourage conservation of energy reserves for the curative response.

Restlessness

Due to organic disease and damage to the central nervous system, or from temperamental factors and the accumulation of nervous energy from worry and stress that cannot be dispersed. Symptoms include:- tension, restlessness, agitation, insomnia and anxiety.
REMEDIES
Arsenicum, Nux vomica, Medorrhinum, Zinc. met.

Retarded Milestones

The causes are variable and careful attention must be given to the history and any investigations felt to be in the patient's best interests. Common problems include:- subnormality, Down's syndrome (mongolism), vitamin or hormonal deficiency diseases, diet and nutritional factors, familial causes, mental illness, infection and chronic disease.

REMEDIES

Baryta carb., Calcarea carb., Medorrhinum, Silicea, Sulphur, Tub. bov.

Retention of Urine

The inability to pass urine, usually due to spasms of the sphincter or a fibrous stricture from earlier disease. In some common cases the cause is due to trauma of the bladder expulsive muscles. Other causes are blockage from a bladder calculus or prostatic disease.

REMEDIES

Cantharis, Causticum, China, Opium, Sabal Serrulata, Thuja.

Rheumatic Fever

The acute generalised allergic condition of young people following a haemolytic *streptococcal* throat infection. The throat is severely infected, the joints inflamed, red and swollen, often involvement of the pericardium leading to pericarditis and inflammation of the heart valves, especially the mitral valve. If scarring occurs there may be mitral stenosis and narrowing in adult years unless the condition is thoroughly treated at the time. A course of penicillin is often recommended

to avoid the risks of cardiac complications and all cases must be under the care of an experienced physician.
REMEDIES
Aconitum, Bryonia, China, Crataegus, Mercurius, Pulsatilla, Rhus tox., Sulphur.

Rheumatism

This is usually muscular in origin from changes in the muscles and tendons acting like a barometer - expanding and contracting with atmospheric pressure and aggravated by damp or cold. Such changes pull on tiny nerve fibres of the tendon and muscle sheath, causing pain. When it occurs in the low back area it produces acute lumbago. It is often chronic because of our damp climate and island conditions and more of a nuisance than anything else. Stress of any kind always aggravates the condition, as does strain and fatigue.
REMEDIES
Bryonia, Causticum, Dulcamara, Medorrhinum, Rhus tox.

Rheumatoid Arthritis

The common acute inflammatory joint condition of unknown origin. It is probably an allergic reaction but this is still unproven. The condition is commoner in females of the 20-40 year age group, than in the male. There is no associated cardiac involvement. Swelling, pain, stiffness with raised temperature, loss of use due to pain with muscle wasting and distortion of joints can occur. Depression of mood is frequent. The condition may resolve completely, or become chronic with joints and movement rigid and fixed from ossification (bony changes within the tendons), fibrosis and distortion.

REMEDIES
Aconitum, Apis, Belladonna, Causticum, Medorrhinum, Natrum mur., Ruta. The patient's constitutional prescription.

Rhinitis

Inflammation of the lining nasal mucosa with thickening and congestion, leading to catarrhal discharge, varying with the type and degree of infection.
REMEDIES
Calcarea, Kali carb., Pulsatilla, Sulphur.

Rhododendron (Rhododendron Chrysanthum)

Mainly a remedy for rheumatic problems with pain and spasm of fibrous and muscular tissue and sensitivity to changes of climate. Also for inflammation of the testicle. All symptoms are:- aggravated by damp, prolonged sitting and inactivity, or an impending thunder storm, and better after the storm has passed. There is relief from movement and exercise.

Rhus Tox (American Poison Ivy)

One of the most useful of all homoeopathic remedies. The mood is one of restlessness irritability and anxiety. It acts on skin, muscle, fibrous tissue around the joints and is of particular value in rheumatic conditions where there is pain, stiffness and incapacity. All symptoms are worse from immobility of any kind, prolonged sitting or sleeping. The skin is red, irritated, swollen with vesicle formation. It is also helpful for Shingles. Cold and damp aggravate the rheumatic pains and stiffness and all symptoms are relieved by heat and movement.

Right-sided Homoeopathic Remedies

Certain remedies have a predisposition for one side of the body and act strongly on problems in these areas. The major right-sided remedies are:-
Colocynth, Dioscorea, Indigo, Lycopodium, Magnesium phos., Naphthaline, Palladium, Tellurium.

Rosa Canina (Dog Rose)

Tincture of ripe hips, first proved by Compton-Burnett. A remedy for chronic bladder and prostate problems, with difficulty and slowness in passing urine.

Rosmarinus Officinalis (Rosemary)

Tincture of the whole plant. One of our most ancient remedies. The main indications are:- alopecia, poor concentration and memory (compare *Lycopodium)*.

Ross, Andrew Christie Gordon. M.D. (1904-1982)

Educated in Glasgow, Ross studied medicine at St. Andrews, working and practising in Glasgow for most of his life. He worked as an enthusiastic homoeopath, following the traditions of his older brother Douglas. A keen golfer, he was also an author and play-wright. Especially he was prolific in his homoeopathic articles with over 200 to his credit in various journals.
Major writings include:
Homoeopathy - An Introductory Study
Arnica, The Amazing Healer
Homoeopathic Green Medicine

Ross, Thomas Douglas. M.D. (1902-1964)

The eminent Scottish homoeopath, educated at Glasgow University. Superintendent and later consultant to the Glasgow Homoeopathic Hospital, he was President of the Faculty from 1962-64. A keen golfer, musician and prolific writer, he had a keen appreciation of the uniqueness of the individual, which contributed to his standing as a physician and prescriber.

Royal, George. M.D. (1853-1926)

The American homoeopath, Professor of Homoeopathic Materia Medica and Therapeutics in the State University of Iowa for 30 years. Also President and chairman of the Council of Medical Education of the American Institute of Homoeopathy, Member of the Hahnemann Medical Association of Iowa and honourary member of the British Homoeopathic Medical Society.
Major writings include:
1918 A Text Book of Materia Medica
1923 A Textbook of the Homoeopathic Theory and Practice of Medicine

Royal London Homoeopathic Hospital

Founded by Quin (see section) in 1844. Initially in Golden Square, it played an important role in its early days during the Cholera epidemic of 1854, when homoeopathic treatments were so successful that the mortality rate for the disease was only 16% compared with 52%, in all other hospitals. There was considerable hostility to homoeopathy at the time and Quin was instrumental in ensuring that these figures were not suppressed and that there was security of practice for the homoeopathic physicians of his time, when attempts were made to outlaw them. The hospital still plays a major role with both in-patient and out-patient clinical work. Homoeopathic doctors are assured of a thorough training over the three year period of qualification, and regular post-graduate meetings and lectures are held. The faculty of the hospital is responsible for the teaching programme and the doctors' bi-annual membership examination. The high standard of teaching and clinical training ensures wide interest, with doctors coming from many countries. At present, the faculty probably offers the best homoeopathic training in the world.

Royal Patronage

Homoeopathy has been very fortunate to have considerable royal support over many years.
H.M. Queen Elizabeth is patron of the Royal London Homoeopathic Hospital and The Queen Mother is patron of the British Homoeopathic Association. There has been a homoeopathic physician appointed to the royal household since Sir John Weir, followed by Dr. Blackie, Dr. Charles Elliott and recently Dr. Ronald Davey.

Ruddock, Edwin Harris. M.D. (1822-1865)

The eminent English homoeopathic practitioner. Trained at Guys and St. Bartholomew's hospitals, he qualified from Edinburgh in 1865. He became Editor of *The Homoeopathic World journal.*
Major writings include:
A Ladies Manual of Home Treatment
Stepping Stones to Homoeopathy and Health

Homoeopathic Vade-Mecum - (his most important work later revised by Wheeler and Clarke)
Consumption and Tuberculosis of the Lungs
Diseases of Infants and Children
A Pocket Manual of Homoeopathic Veterinary Medicine

Rumex Crisp (Yellow Dock)

The extract of the whole flowering plant. Indicated for catarrh, thick, mucus-laden and abundant, mainly from the nasal and respiratory mucosa and always severely congested. Morning diarrhoea is a feature (compare *Sulphur*). The typical skin itching is improved by heat and worse for cold. All symptoms are better for heat and aggravated by cold or the least draught.

Ruta graveolens (Rue)

Titration of the leaves and young flowering buds. A remedy for fibrous tissues and tendons, in particular where there has been recent strain. Tearing, burning pains are common with a sensation of bruising (compare *Arnica*). There is nodular thickening in the tendons and peri-osteal membrane. Also for contractures of tendons as occurs in chronic rheumatic illness, the hand drawn up, fixed in a claw-shape, or the foot permanently flexed and unusable. Particularly the flexor tendons are affected by the contractures *(Causticum)*. It is also an important eye remedy for strain and fatigue with pain or blurring of vision. The remedy has a role in chronic knee and hip problems. All symptoms are worse for cold, damp weather conditions or strain but often relieved by warm rain.

S

Sabadilla (Veratrum Sabadilla)

Tincture of the pulverised seeds and capsule. It is mainly a left-sided remedy, for chronic catarrhal throat conditions, pain travelling to the right side of the throat or body. (compare *Lycopodium)*. The mucous membrane is inflamed, particularly of the mouth, throat and palate, upper respiratory tract. Also for hay fever with sneezing, conjunctivitis and tapeworm. The typical anxiety is of a hysterical nature with disturbance of body image. The patient usually feels chilly, better for warmth and aggravated by the smell of flowers or fruit.

Sabal Serrulata (The Sabal palm)

Tincture of the fruit, it is a specific prostate remedy for congestion and pain with urinary discomfort. Major symptoms are:- a slow, weak stream with hesitancy or blockage of flow and retention. Cystitis and pain during the sexual act are a further indication. It is often used as the mother tincture, or in very low potencies.

Sabina (Savine)

A pelvic remedy for inflammation and bleeding from the rectal or anal regions, uterus and bladder. The area affected is painful and swollen with throbbing, burning pain leading to cystitis, urgency and strangury (spasm). Exhaustion is common. The periods are disturbed, heavy and prolonged with clots and sudden shooting or bearing-down pains. (Compare *Sepia)*. Indicated for threatened abortion of the third month. The remedy is also used for varicose veins and anal warts.

Salicylic Acid

For problems of tinnitus, vertigo and Meniere's disease. The ear noises are variable, a background hum or buzzing, like loud bells, or sometimes high-pitched with dizziness and nausea. The face often feels hot and red.

Salivary glands - problems of

Cysts may develop when a duct becomes blocked, especially the parotid gland. They are often firm, pea-sized, more of a nuisance and unsightly than a risk to health. In some cases they enlarge and then disappear, only to recur again at a later date for no obvious reason.
REMEDIES
Baryta carb., Calcarea carb., Parotidinum, Silicea.

The salivary glands may become infected locally from mumps, or a bacterial infection causing an abscess with pain and swelling.
REMEDIES
Belladonna, Merc. sol., Pyrogenium.

In the elderly, the flow of saliva may become excessive leading to dribbling, in an otherwise healthy person.
REMEDIES
Merc. sol.

There may be a complete absence of flow of saliva, the mouth, tongue and palate dry.
REMEDIES
Bryonia, Lycopodium, Nux moschata.

Salpingitis

Inflammation of the fallopian tubes - either acute or chronic. The commonest causes are bacterial or viral infection, although chronic causes include gonorrhoea and tuberculosis. The cause needs careful diagnosis and treatment, to avoid damage, especially scarring and blockage, because of the dangers of sterility.

REMEDIES

For acute cases: *Aconitum, Arsenicum, Belladonna, Lachesis, Mercurius.*

For chronic cases: *Graphites, Medorrhinum, Sulphur, Thiosinaminum, Tub. bov.*

Salvia (Sage)

Tincture of the fresh leaves and flowers, it is indicated for chronic throat problems with a dry irritating cough or for chronic gum infections discharging pus.

Sambucus Niger (Elder)

A remedy for oppressive states of fear and anxiety, often associated with a high-pitched laryngitis and hoarseness.

Sanguinaria Canadensis (Blood Root)

A right-sided remedy for chronic nasal and throat conditions, including catarrh, bronchitis, hay fever, bronchitis and winter colds. There is general weakness and exhaustion and a tendency to migraine and vomiting. Circulatory problems with hot flushes and palpitations are also common.

Santoninum (Santonin)

A remedy for worm parasitic conditions, especially threadworm, with irritation of the anal area and an itchy nose. Strabismus or squinting is often associated with worms. Also for cataract, vomiting and diarrhoea. There is a chronic cystitis, difficulty in passing water, frequency, nocturnal enuresis (bed wetting).

Sarsaparilla (Smilax)

A bladder remedy for chronic states of weakness and exhaustion. A diagnostic symptom is inability to pass water when standing, but more easily when sitting. Also for bladder stones, the urine thick with sandy deposits, enuresis, passing water frequently at night, gout and chronic constipation.

Scarlet Fever

The acute infection of childhood. The characteristic bright-red rash occurs on covered areas of the body before involving the face and body totally. A sore throat with a raised temperature is usual and in severe cases the kidney is involved. The disease is highly infectious, although in recent years it has followed a more benign course and is seen less frequently than in earlier years, when mortality was high in epidemics. Sporadic cases of the severe form occur but in general they are rare, although they occasionally cause a major complication. Medical care is essential.

REMEDIES

Aconitum, Belladonna, Bryonia, Lachesis, Merc. sol., Rhus tox, Sulphur.

Schizophrenia

The acute psychotic mental illness, marked by withdrawal, isolation, and a break from reality. Delusional thinking with hallucinations and ideas of reference (others are looking and talking about them), is characteristic. It occurs in shy, passive, young people especially when the background is unstable, or there is an intolerable situation. A typical example might be a university student on a maintenance grant, pressured by work, tutor and his family. In some cases, there is a suicidal risk.
REMEDIES
Argentum nit., Aurum met, Medorrhinum, Natrum mur., Stramonium, Sulphur.

Schmidt, Pierre. M.D. (1894-1987)

The eminent homoeopath and teacher. Graduate of Geneva, he saw as a young man his father's chronic enteritis treated effectively by homoeopathy when all else had failed. Years later, in 1918, he experienced the value of the 200 C. potency of *Influenzinum nosodum* during the 'flu epidemic. He learned homoeopathy from Fredericka Gladwin, a pupil of Kent. Schmidt was one of the major forces of homoeopathic principles in both France and Switzerland. Formerly an assistant at the Royal London Homoeopathic Hospital, he knew and worked with Clarke and Weir (see sections). In 1918, he went to Philadelphia to study the principles of the single remedy and high potency prescribing. Founder of the Hahnemann group in Lyon, he worked mainly in research and post-graduate studies. Founder-member of the International League and Honourary President, Schmidt has translated into French some of

Hahnemann's major works. These include his *Materia Medica, Chronic Diseases* and the sixth edition of the *Organon.* He was known for his many papers on philosophy, materia medica and clinical cases throughout a distinguished career. In 1955 at the 200th centenary celebrations of Hahnemann's birth, he gave a lecture on The Legacy of Hahnemann. In 1960 he reported that a veterinary pupil of his had outstanding results in Foot and Mouth disease using the fresh Nosode prepared yearly in the 30c, 200c and M potency with *Nitric acid.*
Major writings include:
1980 Defective Illness

Schuessler, Willhelm Heinrich. M.D. (1898-1921)

The eminent 19th century homoeopathic physician. Born in Germany he studied medicine in both Berlin and Paris. He was founder of the Biochemic system, using twelve basic salts to restore cellular vitality and balance. It is largely an off-shoot of homoeopathy because it attempts to concentrate on cellular activity only and ignores the mentals and overall features and symptoms. Classical theory regards such cellular imbalance as a largely secondary phenomena.
Major writings include:
1880 *The Twelve Tissue Remedies*

Schultz Law

Developed by the experimental physiologists Arndt and Schultz. Working with minute plants and yeasts they found that a small stimuli enhances growth, medium stimuli impedes it and strong stimuli destroy activity. The effect of *Arsenicum* on yeast cells has confirmed this with a weak solution stimulating cellular growth, and a strong solution destroying growth and life. We can equate the homoeopathic potency with a weak stimulating solution to vital energy and responses and a strong solution with the suppressant drugs - destroying life and activity in the area. This is clearly seen after massive doses of an antibiotic, when physiological functioning may take days or weeks, to fully recover.

Sciatica

Pain due to irritation of the sciatic nerve. There is a dull ache in the buttock along the root of the nerve and often referred down the back or side of the thigh and lower limb to the ankle. Causes are variable and include herniation of an intervertebral disc, with severe paralysing symptoms, or a vertebral displacement which requires osteopathic re-alignment. At other times, disease of the spine or pelvis, may irritate the spinal sciatic nerve roots and cause the symptom.
REMEDIES
Aconitum, Arsenicum, Bryonia, Causticum, Chamomilla, Colocynth, Magnesium phos., Nux vomica, Plumbum, Rhus tox., Tellurium.

Scientific Principles of Homoeopathy

Homoeopathy is prescribed by matching the proving, toxicology and clinical pictures of the remedy, to the clinical symptomatology and overall picture of the patient. The assumption by the physician is that, when the remedy-picture matches the patient, there will be a consistent vital reaction in terms of clinical change and symptoms, according to well-established laws of homoeopathic response. This is the essence of homoeopathy and it meets all the criteria of the scientific method, by testing a hypothesis and predicting an outcome in a consistent method of approach.

In the science of aerodynamics, the computer is used extensively. With careful input of data, mathematically sound, it is possible to predict exactly the flight pathway of the next generation of Aerobus - their speed, efficiency, fuel consumption and cost-efficiency. Models can be developed from the computer data to simulate flight pathways and to predict and correct faults which are likely to develop - at a stage where the plane has barely left the drawing board.

However if you feed similar data into the computer, for the weight, size, wing-span and frequency of wing-movement, for the bumble-bee, the computer comes up with the conclusion that it cannot fly. The fault is not in the computer, it lies in the particular form of data supplied, with its inherent limits and boundaries, and when these are exceeded it gives a wrong or negative response. The computer is only designed to evaluate and process the particular type of data which is fed into it. This is the same problem with the common criticism of homoeopathy - that it is not working or valid, because it does not conform to the particular criteria of the double-blind method. Like the computer however, it is designed solely to evaluate its own particular brand of data. Again the fault is not that of homoeopathy, or that it is inconsistent, invalid and unscientific, but lies with the method of evaluation and appraisal of the experimental model. Concepts of double-blind and cross-over experiments are recent innovations and lead to poor results because it is impossible to exactly match one human or group of humans, with another similar group. They just don't exist and 'approximately' is not good enough in this area of prediction and response. These are however purely points of technique and do not relate to a basic scientific method of approach. Much of the recent talk of the value of statistics is in fact, very suspect when considering scientific method, because it can be endlessly manipulated to fit the results and to either validate or invalidate them. They are largely irrelevant to sound scientific methods which in homoeopathy are based on clinical studies and clinical results. The 'scientifics' are often doubly blind themselves - because they fail to see the limitations and bias of their own models and to appreciate the true merits of alternative methods like homoeopathy (which though clinically sound, fails to fit into their own particular brand of data-evaluation and logic).

The major area of criticism of homoeopathy has not been so much about its method or principles, but concerns the use of infinitely small dilutions - beyond the molecular or material limit. The electron microscope has in recent years considerably extended our scope and knowledge of cellular life, functioning and structure to the extent, that most of our physiology and neuro-physics is now being re-written and re-thought.

In war, we now use the single Exocet missile - one dot on a radar screen, fired from something approaching thirty miles away, at a blob on a similar radar screen - yet capable of destroying a battle-ship, which is invisible to the naked eye. It is only deviated from its target and inevitable 'hit' by a smoke-screen of similar radar blobs. Likewise the sub-microscope virus can create devastation in the human organism, once it has gained entry into the physiological soil, with vitality and resistance minimal.

Opium has been used very effectively in medicine for thousands of years and no one has seriously doubted its importance or validity. Yet is only in very recent years that some understanding has emerged as to its mode of action on pain by secreting minute opium-like endorphin at nerve endings within the central nervous system. In a similar way we are only now beginning to understand how homoeopathy works, although its action is beyond doubt. The mode of action of Aspirin as a pain-killer is still not understood - but it can be an effective pain-killer.

The importance of essential trace elements such as:- copper, manganese, cobalt, present in minute amounts, has only recently been fully appreciated and made measurable as new techniques develop - often from such varied fields as space-technology and satellite studies. Similarly vitamins are required in minute quantities to ensure health.

As we enter into the age of nuclear medicine from nuclear war, it is likely that the true significance of the infinitesimal and the single dosage in potency will be more widely appreciated. Homoeopathy, by imprinting its blue-print on the processes of dilution and succussion, energises and organises the solution. But measurable proof is still being researched. Throughout the whole of medicine, scientific proof of a remedy and method, usually lags behind every-day clinical evidence of its efficacy and value for the patient.

We are still awaiting further developments in nuclear medicine to give us the measuring instrument to accurately differentiate and measure our potencies, to record their unique energy patterns and levels of specificity. There have already been several experiments in the past which have shown the stimulant effect of potencies of up to $10^{-17,}$ on algae growth and isolated muscles of the frog's heart. The 6c potency of Phosphorus ($10^{-12)}$ has been shown to measurably regenerate rat liver cells, poisoned with carbon tetrachloride. But homoeopathy is not based or built-up on animal experiments and we await an outcome of confirmation at a more human level.

Such delay in no way detracts from the homoeopathic method or the scientific principles of the approach. The homoeopath is daily extending his patients by the potencies, freeing bound-up static energy to cure disease and at the same time, freeing the patient for a fuller more meaningful life. In many ways it is not for homoeopathy to catch up with science, but science to catch up with homoeopathy.

Sea Sickness

The common problem of motion sickness at sea, worse for inclement weather, another person being ill which acts as a psychological stimulus to vomiting, also the smell of diesel oil.

REMEDIES

Argentum nit., Arnica, Berberis, Cocculus, Nux vom., Petroleum, Tabacum.

Seasonal Factors in homoeopathic prescribing

Many remedies have an optimum sphere or power of action at certain times of the year. This is not easily explainable but it bears a relationship to the time at which the plant flowers are picked for preparation of the tincture and when its intrinsic energy is at a peak. *Pulsatilla* is mainly a spring remedy, *Sabadilla* works best in late spring and early summer. *Sulphur* acts best with the new moon, *M.A.P.* is primarily a late summer and early autumn remedy.

Secale Cornutum (Rye Ergot)

A circulatory remedy for burning pains, the area affected becoming bluish, numb and irritated with a tingling 'pins and needles' discomfort. The toes and fingers may become black and gangrenous. Ulceration may also occur. All symptoms are worse from heat and better for cold air (compare *Sulphur)*. Spasms and convulsions are characteristic with a tendency to bleeding. Also for:- dryness of the skin and mucous membrane with catarrh, paralysis, numbness, sterility and recurrent miscarriage.

Selenium (Red Selenium)

Indicated for general weakness and exhaustion with weight loss, emaciation, chronic laryngitis and paralysis. It also helps depression, alopecia, alcoholism, impotency. There is a tendency to bladder weakness with slight leaking on walking or movement (compare *Causticum)*.

Senecio Aureus (Golden Ragwort)

Mainly a remedy for young women with menstrual problems. The periods are either suppressed or absent or there is excessive colicky pain on the first day. The cause of the missed periods can be a chill, or from continuous overland travelling. Amenorrhoea can also occur in air-hostesses on regular long-haul flights. The remedy is also indicated for:- tuberculosis, chronic catarrh, haemorrhagic tendencies e.g. violent nose bleeds, cystitis, renal failure. There is a typical 'rattling' cough at night.

Sepia Officinalis (Ink of the Cuttlefish)

One of Hahnemann's major anti-psoric remedies and known since antiquity as a medicine for female problems. It is primarily for the tall, thin, rather sallow woman, often strangely indifferent to those around her. It is of value for puerperal depression. The woman is often nervous, moody, irritable, feeling worn-out, totally lacking in joy and incapable of any form of positive response. At the end of the day she feels exhausted, old and dragged down by pain, fatigue and chronic backache. There is frequently a saddle-shaped brown mark across the bridge of her nose. Pelvic pain with uterine prolapse is common - the pains dragging-down in type. Chronic constipation with canine hunger is common and she is always better for quick, brisk movements, such as dancing or walking and worse for thunderstorms.

Sexual Problems

Difficulties are usually psychological in origin with a few exceptions due to hormonal imbalance, or the side-effect of a prescribed drug treatment. The contraceptive 'pill' can frequently diminish libido. Often there is an underlying problem of immaturity or ambivalence to the opposite sex, sometimes dating from earliest years. This needs to be discussed, together with the whole area of sexual fantasy. Whenever possible, limit childish magical thinking and omnipotence, by frank open discussion. There should be no 'secrets' about sex as these form clusters of anxiety which feed any problem areas. The response to homoeopathy in both sexes is very encouraging.

REMEDIES
For frigidity: *Pulsatilla, Graphites, Ignatia, Platina, Onosmodium.*
For 'honeymoon' cystitis: *Staphysagria.*
For impotency: *Argentum nit., Caladium, Selenium Silicea.*
For painful intercourse: *Causticum.*
For premature ejaculation: *Lycopodium, Medorrhinum, Nux vomica.*

Shingles (See section - Herpes Zoster)

Silicea (Silica)

Trituration of the element. A deep acting polycrest remedy for chronic disease. The patient is typically thin and chilly with a profuse, offensive sweat, especially about the feet which feel as if in a 'wet sock' most of the day. There is exhaustion with nervousness and timidity - lacking totally in 'grit', confidence, the ability to see a problem through, staying power and determination. There are many chronic problems of inflammation with pus formation. *Silicea* is often called the 'mother of pus', because every lesion seems to suppurate and discharge pus. Also for occipital (back of the head) headaches, tending to radiate forward to the forehead or over one eye. The skin is typically cracked and infected, the fingers dead white. Every symptom is aggravated by chill and the least cold draught of air. It is also helpful for enuresis (bed wetting).

Simillimum

The homoeopathic remedy that has the power in its original unpotentised toxic state to produce similar symptoms to those of the patient and thereby to relieve them by its action on the vital energy in this same area. According to Hahnemann the simillimum has a natural tendency to form similar symptoms, as in its undiluted state and it is this tendency which allows the patient's symptoms to be unlocked and available to the normal process of resistance and cure which is intrinsic to everyone. Vital energy is bound or blocked by suppressed illness, which creates suppressed energy. The potencies are able to release this trapped energy so that it can find a new and more healthy level of expression and functioning.

Simpson, Sir James Young. (1811-1870)

The eminent Edinburgh Professor of midwifery who first used chloroform in surgery and labour as an anaesthetic. He was teacher and friend of Skinner and Drysdale (see sections). Although not a homoeopath, he nevertheless was in advance of his time in many major areas. He particularly advocated single-remedy prescribing rather than the poly-pharmacy of his time. He had a great influence over Skinner, and paved the way for many of his later contributions. In homoeopathy, single remedy prescribing is one of its major therapeutic principles.

Sinusitis

Inflammation of the mucous membrane of the sinuses, leading to catarrh, discharge and headache - often over one eye with local tenderness over the blocked sinus due to the inflammation.
REMEDIES
Hepar sulph., Kali bich., Pulsatilla, Sulphur.

Skinner, Thomas. M.D. (1825-1906)

The distinguished Edinburgh homoeopath who until the age of fifty was antagonistic to the method - as indeed was at first Hering, and many other eminent early workers. He invented the 'Skinner Machine', a method of preparing high potencies. The original machine is now at the Faculty of Homoeopathy, London. He practised in Liverpool and London, working closely with Clarke and Burnett (see sections). With Lippe in the U.S. he formed the International Hahnemannian Association and was co-editor of *The Organon* journal. Major writings include:
1878 Homoeopathy and Gynaecology

Sleep Problems

This is a common problem which requires careful exploration and prescribing. The cause can be due to noise and the environment, occupation and shift-work, pain, e.g. from arthritis, rheumatism, organic disease, indigestion, hormonal imbalance, or due to an overactive mind and a fearful temperament. Anxiety or depression are often the underlying causes of the sleep problem.

REMEDIES
Aconitum from fear and anxiety.
Arsenicum waking with panic or anxiety after midnight to 1.00 am.
Coffea due to abuse of tea or coffee.
Kali carb. waking with anxiety in the early morning hours 3-5.00 am.
Lachesis from drenching night-sweats.
Lycopodium for an over-active mind, unable to rest or relax.
Nux vomica from dietary indiscretions.
Pulsatilla insomnia due to the heat of the bed.

Sleep Walking (Somnambulism)

When it is persistent, there is usually a deep underlying psychological problem that needs exploring.
REMEDIES
Kali brom., Lycopodium, Stramonium.

Snoring

A common problem. The underlying causes include:- polyps, adenoids, chronic throat infections or catarrh.
REMEDIES
Kali bich., Opium.

Sol

Potentisation of lactose powders exposed to sunlight. It is useful for problems aggravated by heat or the sun's rays, with intolerance to sunlight of any kind. This may occur in sensitive skin conditions or photophobia. Also for sunstroke and allergies worse for heat and sun.

Solidago Virga Aurea (Golden Rod)

A remedy for chronic conditions of the renal organs, particularly with low renal output and renal colic. Also for dysuria and urinary retention (compare *Natrum mur.* and *Causticum).*

Spasm

Spasm can occur in any part of the body wherever there is smooth muscle. The major symptoms are pain, interference with normal physiological functioning and often anxiety. The cause may be indigestion, allergy, or apprehension and fear. Other causes are:- irritation (from a stone or calculus), infection, dietary factors, or allergy.

REMEDIES

Aconitum when due to fear.

Causticum spasm of the larynx.

Cicuta spasm of the throat and glottis (compare *Drosera* and *Ignatia).*

Cuprum met. spasm of the calf muscles and feet.

Nux vomica spasm of the stomach.

Phosphorus spasm of the bronchial tubes.

Spigelia (Pinkroot)

Tincture of the whole plant. It is mainly a left-side remedy. There is severe neuralgia of the face, neck and shoulders, aggravated by cold air, touch, or movement. (compare *Belladonna, Colchicum, Kalmia, Platina, Nux vomica.*) Also palpitations with Angina.
(compare *Cactus and Latrodectus).*

Spongia Tosta

An important cardiac remedy with anxiety, palpitations, fear of death, depression and cardiac pain. There may be valvular disease of the heart with shortness of breath, asthma, cardiac enlargement and weakness. Also for laryngitis with hoarseness and dryness of the throat. All symptoms are worse for sleep (Compare *Lachesis)*, better for sitting up and for warm drinks. Any breathlessness is aggravated by lying flat.

Sprains

Traumatic injury to the tendons as a result of a fall or strain. The tendons are stretched, bruised, or torn in severe cases with pain, bruising, incapacity and stiffness. Swelling of the area may be marked due to a haematoma (bleeding into local tissues).
REMEDIES
Arnica, Bellis per., Calc. carb., Kali carb. Sulphur.

Stammering

The common stutter. A nervous problem of speech, mainly psychological in origin. It is aggravated by new situations or pressure of any kind. Treatment is often best when combined with regular speech-therapy, especially in severe cases.
REMEDIES
Belladonna, Mercurius, Stramonium.

Stannum (Tin)

There is increasing weakness, weight-loss and exhaustion. The patient is pale and withdrawn, with no interest, due to a near-collapsed state. Also for severe neuralgia and laryngeal hoarseness. There is chronic catarrh with a thick, yellowish mucous discharge, also leucorrhea, the discharge thick and creamy-yellow.

Stapf, Ernest. M.D. (1788-1860)

The German homoeopath, born in Nuremburg who was the earliest of Hahnemann's pupils and a disciple throughout his life, also a close friend of Quin (see section). He studied and worked in homoeopathy as early as 1811, assisting Hahnemann with the *Materia Medica Pura* and working with the limited repertory of the early days. Like Hahnemann, he was ridiculed and often persecuted by his colleagues for his viewpoint, although later considered to be a most respected and serious physician. He was one of the earliest provers of Hahnemann's original group and worked with him in proving some 32 remedies. He became founder and first editor of the very first homoeopathic journal *Archiv. fur die Homoepathirsche Heilkunst*, (1822-39). A staunch believer in the harmful effects to the patient of coffee, wine, and tobacco, he may have been the first appointed royal homoeopathic physician. In 1835 he became visiting physician to the royal household, having previously carried out homoeopathic treatments by letter.

Major writings include:
1846 Additions to the Materia Medica Pura

Staphysagria (Stavesacre)

One of the most valuable remedies wherever there is anger or irritability, with indignation and buried resentments. Pain is severe, tearing and stitch-like. Also for cystitis from trauma or injury, with bruising. It is helpful for prostate problems and impotence, but especially useful after surgery, for pain around the incision. Resentment and anger is characteristic.

Sterility

This is often a complex problem which needs thorough investigation to ascertain the causes. They may lie with either partner, and it is important to know the roots of the problem and whether there is scarring of the tubes from an earlier infection, or if the sperm count is low, (as may follow adult mumps). It is important that the homoeopath works closely with the gynaecologist.
REMEDIES
For chronic scarring and blockage of the fallopian tubes following infection or operation, consider *Graphites, Silica, Thiosinaminum.*
For diminished sperm count, consider *Lycopodium, Sepia, Silicea.*

Sticta (Lungwort)

Tincture of the fresh plant. It acts primarily upon mucous membrane of the respiratory tract, with bronchial catarrh. The nasal secretions are dry and difficult to expel with little secretion. There are recurrent colds and chronic rheumatic problems. All symptoms are worse for lying down and often aggravated during the night.

Stonham, Thomas. M.D. (1858-1903)

The homoeopathic physician and co-author of *A Manual of Homoeo-therapeutics.*

Storage of homoeopathic remedies

Homoeopathic remedies keep indefinitely without losing strength or efficacy, provided they are stored in a dry, cool, air-tight glass container. This is infinitely preferable to plastic storage bottles, because of chemical impurities present in such containers. The glass bottles should be clean and not have been used to store either homoeopathic or conventional remedies in the past. They should be stored away from any substance which could neutralise them, e.g. camphor, menthol, perfume.

Stramonium (Thorn Apple)

Recommended for states of acute mental excitement, confusion, delirium with loss of control or violent tendencies. There is manic excitement with a tendency to destructive impulses, also delusional beliefs with hallucinations. Convulsions may occur, either epileptic or hysterical in origin. Also for puerperal psychosis with violence and acute mania, suicidal impulses, 'stroke', loss of consciousness, meningitis with excitement or restlessness.

'Stroke'

The acute cerebral catastrophe, usually due to a cerebral haemorrhage, spasm or thrombosis. If severe, there is loss of consciousness, fixed dilated pupils, heavy, snoring-breathing and weakness of one limb. There is often a history of raised blood-pressure. Medical care is essential, hospitalisation when severe.

REMEDIES

Aconitum, Arnica, Opium, Stramonium. Rescue remedy (Bach) can also be given.

Strophanthus Hispidus (Kombe Seed)

Mainly indicated for:- cardiac irregularity with a variable pulse, palpitations and shortness of breath on effort. Especially of value where there is a history of chronic smoking or alcoholism (compare *Nux Vomica).*

Styes

The common localised infection of the eyelids - either acute and clearing completely or recurrent. In some cases it is a chronic condition, the stye remaining for many months and never really healing. Irritation is its main feature.The cause is often due to scratching or rubbing of the area.

REMEDIES

Baryta carb., Calcarea carb., Hepar sulph., Pulsatilla, Silicea, Staphysagria.

Suicidal Impulses

Suicidal thoughts of a passing nature are common and usually no more than a temporary idea or dramatic fantasy which is never acted upon or seriously considered. Suicide is always an act of aggression. In some cultures the most aggressive act conceivable is to commit suicide on an enemy's doorstep. It is no longer rare in our stressful, pressurised, often alienated society and the thought may become a threat and a reality at any age, especially when part of a schizophrenic or depressive illness. In severe depression, threats must be taken seriously, treatment under the care of a physician having a good rapport and understanding with the patient and a natural sympathy for the problem. If anyone reading this book, is desperate and isolated, you can always obtain help by contacting by phone, the nearest branch of The Samaritans, at any time - day or night. Their address is in the telephone book, or the operator will give you the number.

REMEDIES

Argentum nit., Alumina, Aurum met, Capsicum, Naja, Natrum mur., Natrum sulph., Nux. vomica.

Sulphur (Flowers of Sulphur)

The most important of Hahnemann's anti-psora remedies for chronic disease. Body-shape is varied, but frequently thin, bent-over, red-faced, untidy and unhealthy-looking. The patient takes little exercise and is chronically tired and exhausted. Intolerant of heat he is warm-blooded and needs few clothes or covering on the coldest day. The skin is typically unhealthy and infected with a variety of discharging sores and rashes, often of a thick, offensive nature. A morning diarrhoea typically drives him out of bed and the stool is usually offensive. Fats are craved and the butter is always spread thickly. Water or bathing aggravates all symptoms. Flashes of heat, hot-flushes, drenching sweats and weariness are characteristic, the mind full of plans and projects, but always unrealizable or unrealistic and rarely carried through to any conclusion. It is also a remedy for chronic problems where there is little or no response to well-indicated homoeopathic prescribing.

Sulphuric Acid

A remedy for depression combined with exhaustion and near collapse. The patient is restless and always in a hurry (compare *Medorrhinum)*. Tremor is associated with weakness and chronic skin problems, with boils, bed-sores, ulceration and chronic indigestion. A sore cracked mouth is characteristic, ulcerated and infected at the corners with bleeding (Compare *Nitric acid, Silicea)*. Also for Pyorrhoea, the gums unhealthy and infected, contributing to depression and a lowered vital resistance. It is mainly a right-sided remedy.

Sunstroke

In a sensitive person, this can be a very dangerous or fatal condition when exposure has been severe or prolonged. It may have been to the sun's rays directly, or indirectly the result of exposure to high temperatures. Both can be perilous if excessive. The main symptoms are:- a throbbing headache, weakness, collapse, vomiting, sweating and redness, loss of consciousness, fits or paralysis. Hospitalisation is essential in severe cases.

REMEDIES

Aconitum, Belladonna, Bryonia, Glonoin, Pulsatilla.

Repeat the remedy every few minutes until there is a response.

Suppression

Any form of suppression - of the person, opinion, or symptoms is against basic homoeopathic principles and often damaging. The only exception is an overwhelming infection, after an operation, when pain is severe and unbearable, or in a terminal illness, and even in the latter, only pain and not awareness should be blocked. Homoeopathy anticipated psychoanalytic insight, by nearly a century, when it warned against the dangers of suppression. It can never lead to cure and at best only relieves for temporary periods. Suppression of symptoms, means suppression of the vital response, of energy and ultimately of individuality. Many of our major modern conventional synthetic drugs - steroids, tranquillisers and antibiotics act totally by this means, suppressing reactions, natural response and resistance. Suppression of symptoms never gets to the roots of a condition or the cause of an illness - either physical or psychological. The problem is quite simply driven 'underground' where it festers, becomes chronic and is in danger of re-appearing in a new more resistant form, sometimes in a deeper organ or new area of the body and this time much more difficult to treat. Homoeopathy aims to stimulate the vital reaction of the individual and the organism, seeing this as the only true and curative pathway for treatment and cure. Prolonged suppression over the years, is one of the major causes of chronic disease in our society.

Swan, Samuel. M.D. (1814 - 1893)

The American homoeopath and innovator, who first prepared the nosode *Lyssin* from the saliva of a rabid dog as a prophylactic treatment for rabies. He was a colleague of Boericke, Skinner and Fincke (see section) and is best known for his work on the nosodes. He described a first proving of *Syphilinum* in 1880, also developing the nosodes *Lac Caninum* and *Tuberculinum* (from Tuberculosis sputum).

Sycosis (Fig Wart Disease)

One of the major miasms of chronic disease postulated by Hahnemann. It is thought to be due to a previously suppressed gonorrhoeal illness acting as an inherited sub-clinical parasite and undermining health, resistance and energy. The major symptoms are int the skin and take the form of multiple cauliflower-like warts, particularly common in the anal-genital area. Chill on the warmest day is characteristic. *Thuja* and *Nitric ac.* are major sycotic remedies for this miasm.

Sycotic Co. (Paterson)

The bowel nosode. This is a catarrhal remedy acting on mucous membrane throughout the body. Irritability is the key-note mentally, also of the mucous and synovial membranes. Pale and puffy under the eyes, anaemic looking, nervous tension is also characteristic, together with a variety of catarrhal symptoms anywhere in the body. There are many digestive difficulties, also diarrhoea, conjunctivitis, nasal catarrh, deafness, tonsillitis or a sore throat. Also for leucorrhoea, asthma or cystitis with painful spasms, or other renal problems e.g. nephritis or pyelitis. The angles of the mouth, nose and anal area are often cracked, sore and ulcerated. The tongue is fissured and there is an aversion to eggs.

Symphoricarpus Racemosa (Snowberry)

Tincture of the fresh berries, it is a remedy for severe retching and nausea e.g. vomiting of pregnancy, which may be constant throughout the day and night. There is complete lack of interest in food.

Symphytum (Comfrey)

The ancient remedy for deep-seated pains of bones and of assistance whenever there is delay in healing and the uniting of fractures.

Symptoms

That which is experienced by the patient personally as the expression of his malaise. All symptoms are seen by the homoeopath as a healthy vital reaction and struggle towards balance, the individual response to underlying imbalance and dis-ease. Symptoms are not the cause of the illness, but only the visible external manifestation of internal malaise, often dating back over several weeks or months. The absence or weakness of a symptom-response is of more concern to the homoeopath than its presence, reflecting severely limited resistance and vitality. Symptoms are the body's attempts to regain homoeostasis and cure and this quite vital reaction-of-cure needs conserving. It is the underlying *meaning* of the symptoms that needs treatment rather than the symptoms themselves. Simple eradication is undesirable and not in the patient's best, long-term, interests. Homoeopathy always takes an overall viewpoint and the totality of symptoms into account when prescribing.

Symptomatic Treatment

The treatment and relief of symptoms only, by conventional allopathic means, is short-term thinking and only rarely justifiable. The short-term gain does nothing to understand or treat the underlying causes, and it is often a major factor in recurrent disease and the need for constant re-prescribing. Stronger remedies have the dual danger of side-effects and suppression of symptoms, at the expense of cure.

Syncope (Fainting)

The common problem of brief loss of consciousness, often from emotional causes and sometimes recurrent.
REMEDIES
Aconitum when provoked by fear.
Carbo veg. for collapse and fainting from weakness and exhaustion.
China for fainting at the sight of blood.
Ignatia due to emotion, especially from grief and loss, or fear of it.
Pulsatilla for recurrent fainting at the least emotional situation, or from heat.
Veratrum Alb. fainting from pain or emotion - the patient deathly pale in a cold sweat and seemingly about to succumb.
Give the remedy in the 6c potency every few minutes until recovery occurs. A few drops of the potency in water on the tongue, is the most convenient form of application for syncope.

Syphilinum

The syphilis nosode prepared from infected serous exudate (discharge) of the primal chancre (local infection), and made into potency by serial dilutions. First suggested by Lux in 1830. Swan (see section) carried out the initial provings and published the results fifty years later in 1880. The main indications are:- chronic conditions, a history of miscarriage, failure to thrive, and chronic varicose ulcers. Mental symptoms are marked with avoidance- behaviour towards others which may take a phobic form with obsessional fear of contact, infection or 'germs', exhaustion and depression. The patient is often noisy, difficult, stubborn at times, tearful, opposing, varying in mood but especially prone to hand-washing, with mannerisms, tics and nervous mannerisms. Insomnia is characteristic, with all symptoms worse at night or for sea air (compare *Natrum mur.)*. There is typical pain in the tibia or long bones, often at night and a thin, prematurely aged look. The teeth are poor, deformed, notched and cracked. Also for arteriosclerosis, urinary weakness, impotence, genital irritation, leucorrhoea, the discharge greenish and offensive.

T

Tabacum (Tobacco)

Tincture of the fresh plant and a remedy for nausea with pallor, cold sweats and prostration. Also for travel or pregnancy sickness, convulsions, oedema of the soft palate, vertigo. All symptoms are worse for heat (Compare *Pulsatilla)* and better for lying down, darkness and sleep.

Tachycardia

An increase in the heart rate. The normal pulse rate is 72 beats per minute. In tachycardia the rate is increased to 150 or 200 beats per minute. Causes include emotion, infection, toxic or poisonous causes, excesses of tea or coffee, stimulant drugs, allergy, side-effects of drugs, degeneration of the cardiac conducting pathways.
REMEDIES
Crataegus, Lycopus virg., Spigelia, Tarantula hisp.

Taking the remedies

The homoeopathic medicine is mainly on the surface of the tablet or pill. It is important that whenever possible they should not be handled except to a minimum, to avoid neutralising them by perfume or foodstuff on the hands, or by handling generally. The remedies should be taken with an interval of 20-30 minutes, either before or after food, unless there are specific instructions to this effect from the physician. Strong food or drink including coffee, tea, mint, alcohol, should not be taken within half an hour of the remedy.

Tamus Communis (Black Bryony)

One of the most powerful remedies for chilblains with painful itching and redness. It is often used in low potency or as mother tincture.

Tapeworm

The solitary parasitic worm intestinal condition, now relatively rare in European countries due to improved hygiene and preventive practice. Its origin is from infected uncooked beef or pork. Symptoms are:- abdominal pain, weight-loss and segments of the worm in the stool. Isolated causes can still occur and careful diagnosis is essential.
REMEDIES
Calcarea carb., Sabadilla, Sepia, Silicea, Spigelia, Sulphur.

Tarantula Cubensis (Cuban Tarantula)

A remedy for severe burning pains with abscess formation and collapse. Also for anthrax infection. The face is violet, or there is pallor, cold sweating, a sinking sensation, emaciation, shortness of breath and air hunger. Both legs and ankles are swollen. Also for shock and a remedy for the most desperate conditions with lack of response or vitality of reaction (compare *Carbo veg., Veratrum alb.).*

Tarantula Hisp (Spanish Tarantula)

Indicated for states of severe violent restlessness and extreme destructive behaviour. There are burning pains of the limbs with weakness and similar symptoms in the rectum and anus. All symptoms are aggravated by cold and damp. It is indicated for severe mental conditions of hysteria, psychosis, manic excitement. Bright colours and music often aggravate the symptoms. Destructiveness and tearing of clothes is frequent, with jerking movements of the head, agitation, chronic indigestion and flatulence. Other symptoms are:- shooting pains in the uterus and vagina, diarrhoea with blood, spasms of the bladder, prostatitis, pruritus (itching), palpitations. The pulse is rapid and irregular. The key-note is:- irritation, congestion, burning pains in any part of the body, with uncontrollable impulses to violence.

Taraxacum Officinalis (Dandelion, 'Pee-in-the-bed')

The main indications are hepatitis - the liver enlarged and tender, deficient in functioning. There is intolerance of any form of touch or pressure. Also for enuresis.

Taste - loss of

This may accompany a severe cold or 'flu, with associated nasal catarrh and throat congestion affecting the mucosa and inhibiting the taste sensitivity of the tongue's surface. The condition may become chronic.
REMEDIES
Calcarea for chronic problems everything tastes generally sour and unpalatable.
Merc. sol. the tongue is dirty and offensive with thick yellow coating.
Natrum mur. following a cold or 'flu.
Nux vom. there is a generalised sour acid taste whatever is taken, worse in the morning. The tongue has a thick white coating, aggravated by alcohol or smoking.

Pulsatilla due to general congestion - everything has an earthy taste to it.
Sulphur for chronic problems, the food tastes vinegary or of blood.

Teeth

Thorough regular cleaning and flossing are essential for healthy teeth together with dental hygiene and regular prophylactic check-ups to ensure that problems are detected early or avoided. The diet and quality of nutrition is often the key to healthy dental development. Sweet, sugar-rich refined foods should be avoided. Sweets should not be given as a reward to encourage a young child to behave or conform. Decayed or badly-placed teeth blocking the emergence of new ones, must be removed. A root abscess must be drained whenever diagnosed, because of the narrowness of the dental canal and the risk of infection spreading. It should not be just sealed-off under a dressing and local antibiotic before the pus has fully drained from the area.
REMEDIES
For caries and unhealthy dental development: *Calcarea carb., Calcarea phos., Kreosotum, Phosphorus, Silicea.*
For acute toothache: *Aconitum, Belladonna, Chamomilla, China, Coffea, Magnesium carb., Nux vom., Plantago, Selenium, Spigelia, Staphysagria.*
Often the constitutional prescription is required to stimulate healthier dental growth and vitality.

Teething Problems (of the infant)

The commonest symptoms are:- irritability and gum soreness, the child constantly wanting something in his mouth. Problems are most acute from the age of a year when the four bicuspids emerge after the incisors.
REMEDIES
Aconitum there is fear and restless agitation.
Belladonna for a red face, raised temperature and crying when examined or touched.
Calcarea carb. teething and the growth milestones are retarded. For a flabby child with forehead sweating.
Chamomilla the child is irritable and dislikes being put down.
China is useful where an irritating cough is associated.
Drosera the cough is dry and goes on to vomiting.
Merc. sol. should be considered for a child covered in sweat and with profuse, offensive salivation.

Tellurium

Introduced by Hering in 1850, it is a remedy for chronic skin problems especially ringworm of the face and body. Chronic infection is widespread and discharges pus (compare *Sulphur)*. Also for middle ear infection with a thick offensive purulent discharge. Sweating is offensive *(Silicea)*. There is intolerance of the least touch or pressure.

Tendonitis

The inflammatory condition of painful tendons after excessive strain or unaccustomed usage. Swelling, pain, spasm, aching with a bruised sensation is common. Rest, firm strapping or support, avoidance of fatigue in

the area, with the appropriate remedy usually clears the condition in a few days. Local heat is often beneficial.
REMEDIES
Arnica, Rhus tox., Ruta.

Tension States

The common psychological state of anxiety, restlessness, muscular aching, pain, spasm of the stomach or back, palpitations. Panic is often a feature. Discussion and the frank expression of any particular areas of anxiety is essential. However, there is often nothing specific and the tension is a re-emergence of long-standing problems. Physical symptoms of diarrhoea or indigestion need careful attention to exclude an organic problem and must always form part of the totality when selecting the remedy. A tension state should never be prescribed for on the mentals alone and consideration should equally be given to any physical symptoms.
REMEDIES
Arsenicum, Gelsemium, Ignatia, Lycopodium, Natrum mur., Pulsatilla, Sepia.

Terebinth (Oil of Turpentine)

Tincture of the rectified oil, it is predominately a kidney remedy. There are:- unbearable burning pains with irritation, haematuria (blood in the urine), dragging pains in the kidney area, as from nephritis. Also for cystitis with strangury (pain and spasm at the end of the urinary flow). Little urine is passed and there is congestion of the mucous membrane throughout the body with irritation in the areas affected. The remedy is closely related to *Berberis, Cantharis, Thuja.*

Terrain of the Patient

The 'soil' or terrain of the patient refers to the concept that all illness is a combination of diseased physiology with increased susceptibility, diminished resistance and lack of vital energy. The usual 'cause' of disease is a miasm in chronic disease, or such internal irritants as toxins, parasites or anything that undermines the healthy functioning of the part affected. Bacteria, mites, tics and viral agents are seen, as the natural symbiotic inhabitants of our overall environment. When the terrain is weakened and made more susceptible, they cease to live in symbiosis with us. Under such conditions they may actively invade and undermine tissue-functioning leading to infection, inflammation, tumour or abscess formation, but only *after* the physiological terrain has been undermined. One of the major undermining factors is undoubtedly psychological stress or shock with nutritional neglect or abuse coming a close second. Stress can lower the sperm count of the most virile donor within hours - such is its depth of action on vitality.

Terminal Conditions

The homoeopathic remedy has an important role to play in terminal conditions and can relieve or lessen symptoms and their effect, upon the patient's peace of mind. It can 'smooth the way', and allow a paticnt to dic with dignity, yet retain awareness and equanimity. The homoeopathic remedy is not curative here because of lack of vital energy and there is usually a limited response to the 'local' 6c or 3x potencies. It is the higher potencies which are most valuable, especially the 30c and 200c. These can often make the patient wonderfully calm, serene and relaxed so that they need far fewer pain-killers and opiates. Tension, anticipation and worry is also relieved. In some cases, the higher potencies give a marked, albeit temporary relief from symptoms, for a period of several weeks or months. Naturally this does not always occur and each patient must be seen, according to the overall unique picture and the extent and length of time of the illness.

Teste, Alphonse. M.D. (1814-1888)

The French homoeopath who published in 1844 *A Practical Manual of Animal Magnetism,* containing an exposition of the methods employed in producing magnetic phenomena and its application to the treatment and cure of disease. (Translated by Dr. Spillan).
Major writings include:
1854 *The Homoeopathic Materia Medica* (Tr. Hempel)
A Homoeopathic Treatise of Diseases of Children

Testicular Problems

These should always be treated by a physician to ensure careful diagnosis and treatment. The common problem of undescended testicle must be corrected surgically, if the potencies fail to elicit a positive response.
REMEDIES
Aurum met., Pulsatilla.

Hydrocele or fluid around the testicular sac, is a less urgent problem and seen commonly. The origin is sometimes associated with a history of tuberculosis.
REMEDIES
Pulsatilla, Tub. bov.

Orchitis or inflammation of the testicle may be a complication of mumps - one of the commoner causes.
REMEDIES
Merc. sol., Parotidinum, Pulsatilla, Spongia, Thuja.

Tetanus

Severe infection leading to septicaemia, which may follow tetanus contamination of a dirty wound or fracture. The wound must be carefully cleaned with *Calendula* and any foreign material removed. When in doubt, or the wound heavily contaminated with soil or dirty foreign matter, give the specific anti-tetanus vaccine.
REMEDIES
Arnica, Cicuta virosa, Hypericum, Ledum, Merc. sol.

Teucrium Marum (Cat-thyme)

A remedy for chronic sinus problems and nasal catarrh. Loss of smell is characteristic.

Theridion (The orange spider of Curacao)

For oversensitivity and excitement to any stimulus with hysterical behaviour or depression. All symptoms are aggravated by noise, including the chronic nausea and severe pains. Also for:- emaciation, fainting, chill and headache from the forehead backwards towards the base of the skull, worse for the least noise. It is often indicated for tuberculosis, chronic catarrh, morning sickness from gastric catarrh, nausea of pregnancy and of emotional origin, seasickness, weakness, impotence.

Threadworm

Common in children, the minute parasite can spread throughout the family and frequently involves the parents, who also experience the typical symptoms of anal irritation, worse at night. Often the fine white, cotton-wool threadworm can be seen on the stools, confirming the diagnosis. Itching of the tip of the nose is a common symptom, also irritation, insomnia, crying during sleep, grinding the teeth, weight and appetite loss, vomiting with thirst. There is nearly always increased general nervousness. In every case, the nails should be carefully cut back short and kept scrupulously clean. Personal hygiene must be at a high level to avoid constant re-infection.

REMEDIES

Aconitum for the earliest cases.

Belladonna is helpful for night-terrors or nightmares.

Cina for nasal and anal irritation.

Merc. sol. for long-standing problems, resistant to cure.

Nux vomica is indicated for teeth-grinding at night.

Thlaspi Pursa Pastoris (Shepherd's Purse)

An unusual remedy, indicated for disordered menstrual conditions where there is an intermittent flow - the periods occurring on alternative months.

Throat Sore

The condition may involve the soft tissues at the back of the throat causing a localised pharyngitis, or due to an inflammation of the vocal chords (laryngitis) and causing hoarseness. The condition may be localised or diffuse, sometimes involving the whole throat area.

In viral conditions, or when due to cold or 'flu, the temperature may remain normal. It can also be due to over-use of the throat and voice.

REMEDIES

Aconitum for acute cases, with restless fever, anxiety and a burning sensation in the throat.

Belladonna the throat is bright-red, the patient lying motionless, the pain aggravated by swallowing.

Merc. sol. for severe infections with pus formation and profuse sweating.

Phytolacca the throat is purple, swallowing painful.

Lachesis is similar but often left-sided.

Also consider *Arnica, Bryonia, Natrum mur., Pulsatilla* (the latter for strain from over-use).

Thrush

The common genital infection with the Candida Albicans fungal yeast organism which thrives in warm moist areas of the body. It can occur in adults and children and may be persistent. It occurs in males, but is usually non-symptomatic. The male may however act as a carrier. Most symptoms occur in the female, with a white or yellow thick, or clear, but often curdy discharge. The vaginal discharge often has a slight odour, but where the condition is persistent or chronic, this may become offensive. An itchy irritation of the vaginal and vulval area is common, the area affected red, usually due to scratching. It is a frequent side-effects of taking antibiotics or after steroids.

REMEDIES

Alumina, Borax, Graphites, Kreosotum, Merc. sol., Nitric ac., Pulsatilla, Sepia, Sulphur.

Thuja Occidentalis (Tree of Life)

Hahnemann's major remedy for Sycotic miasm states and chronic disease. The typical constitution is usually thin and unhealthy-looking, with profuse offensive sweating over the whole body. Fig-warts and thickened skin areas occur on the hands or feet, but especially in the anal-genital region. These have a tendency to itch, split or bleed. There may also be flattened multiple brownish warts or markings. Also for shingles with vesicle formation or post-shingles neuralgic pains, or any illness that has commenced after vaccination. Also for bladder problems such as cystitis, urethritis and ovarian pain on ovulation. The mental state is one of irritability with bizarre delusional ideas and jealousy (compare *Lachesis*). There is an odd but diagnostic conviction that the body is made of glass and will break, or a live animal is inside the abdomen, or there are localised headaches - as if a nail has been driven through the skull.

Thyroidinum (Thyroid extract)

For slow retarded states, with fluid retention and oedema, exophthalmic goitre (protrusion of the eyeballs), chronic constipation, cardiac symptoms, especially angina or tachycardia. The skin is dry and cool. Also for:- psoriasis, alopecia, nocturnal enuresis. fibroid tumours of the breast or uterus, heavy periods.

Tics

The common psychological nervous problem with involuntary movements of any part of the body, aggravated by an unfamiliar situation or increase of psychological pressure. 'Live flesh' or tics occur around the lower eyelid area when there has been a build-up of tension or fatigue, the body unable to 'let go' or relax adequately. Homoeopathy combined with discussion and reassurance usually resolves the problem.

REMEDIES

Agaricus, Arsenicum, Natrum mur., Nux vomica.

Time Modalities

Certain remedies, especially the broader and deep-acting polycrests, have a specific time when they are most active with an aggravation of symptoms. Knowledge of such modalities, is of help to prescribing and gives a check on accuracy. Examples are:- *Arsenicum* midnight to 1.00 am., *Kali carb.* 3.00-5.00 am., *Lycopodium* 4.00-8.00 pm. *Natrum mur.* 9.00-11.00 am.

Tongue - problems of

The appearance and condition of the tongue gives an important clue to the overall health of the individual. A thick yellow-coated tongue may indicate chronic indigestion and a remedy such as *Nux vomica.* A more white coating indicates *Bryonia.* Where the coating is yellow and offensive, consider *Mercurius.* Inflammation and ulceration may be caused by trauma, the tongue bitten in an accident or during an epileptic fit. Give *Arnica.* Where the sides of the tongue are painful and swollen, as after an insect bite, use *Apis.* An acute infection (glossitis) may require *Belladonna,* the tongue bright red, with pain and burning discomfort. Where the redness and soreness is at the tip, use *Rhus tox.*

Tonsillitis

Inflammation of the tonsils with pain, a raised temperature, swelling, tender local lymph glands of the neck region. Exhaustion, vomiting and severe discomfort is common. Swallowing is usually painful.
REMEDIES
Aconitum, Baryta carb., Belladonna, Hepar sulph., Merc. sol., Phytolacca, Silicea, Sulphur.

Torticollis (Wry neck)

The common condition of stiff neck, usually rheumatic in origin from exposure to chill, cold air or a draught, provoking spasm of local muscles. It is nearly always short-lasting and clears up spontaneously in a few days with warmth, protection and the appropriate remedy. If it fails to resolve quickly, it may be psychological in origin or has a different deeper cause which needs investigating.
REMEDIES
Argentum nit., Causticum, Dulcamara, Natrum mur, Nux vom., Merc. sol.

Totality of the homoeopathic approach

The basis of all homoeopathy. In the *Organon* (para. 7), Hahnemann describes the totality of symptoms as the outer image of the individual, reflecting the inner essence of the disease and the disturbed vital (life) force. Totality of approach takes into account the outer complaints or symptoms and the inner depths, with a detailed appraisal of the underlying causative factors. The patient's relationship with the doctor and the degree of rapport established is often important. The homoeopathic approach also takes note of the spoken as well as the unspoken communications, the subjective as well as the objective impressions, the way the symptoms are described and presented, the appearance, expression and associations. The mind with all the feelings, motivations, pain, and attitudes is very important, but also the type of work, clothes, the gait, body-odour, any mannerisms. Each and every aspect - both physical and mental, contributes to an overall totality of impression and fact.

The majority of the patient's symptoms must fit the remedy and odd isolated symptoms can be ignored, once they have been considered within the diagnostic framework. The concept of totality expresses a whole - including the symptoms, the simillimum, the cause, the role of suppression, or a miasm. Eventually the totality comes to express far more, than its component parts taken in isolation.

Tracheitis

Inflammation of the trachea, with soreness and pain. There is often a sharp cough, raised temperature, or hoarseness and laryngitis. It is a frequent complication of the common cold and needs careful treatment to avoid pulmonary involvement such as bronchitis.

REMEDIES

Aconitum, Belladonna, Bryonia, Hepar sulph., Mercurius, Sulphur.

Travel Sickness

The problem of motion sickness is especially a difficulty for the young, although it can occur at any age. See heading Sea-Sickness. It is common in a sensitive nervous child and always aggravated by reading. Nausea, sweating, salivation, vomiting are common, with an overall sense of malaise.

REMEDIES

Cocculus, Natrum mur., Nux vomica, Pulsatilla.

Treatment - aims of homoeopathic

In all cases, the aim is simply and solely to restore the person to full normal balance and health. The symptoms or dis-ease manifestations are not the prime concern of the homoeopath, nor should they be for the patient. Symptoms are indications and guide-lines to prescribe and should not distract the homoeopath from his basic role, of restoring the patient's vital energy and well-being. Once this is restored and corrected, the external manifestations fall into place and perspective, as the blocked energy flows and functions again.

Trillium Pendulum (White Beth-Root)

Primarily a gynaecological remedy, it is especially indicated for uterine haemorrhage and recurrent miscarriage of the third month. It has also a valuable therapeutic role in menopausal flooding and fibroids.

Trituration

The unique process, discovered by Hahnemann, of making soluble for dilution and potency substances which are normally considered insoluble. Examples are *Aurum met., Silicea,* or any of the other metals or minerals. During the initial trituration the substance is mixed and ground up with lactose powder. This process is repeated, mixing and grinding, until the substance becomes soluble - usually at the third trituration. Each trituration is considered a centesimal-equivalent and the next dilution and succussion in liquid, forms the fourth centesimal 4c potency.

Tuberculinum (Tuberculinum bovinum)

The subject of a detailed monogram and research by Dr. Compton Burnett and one of his most important contributions. The nosode is prepared from tuberculous glandular material of infected cattle. It is a most important remedy acting deeply on problems of chronic disease which no other remedy can fully reach. Typical indications are:- a dry, irritating, recurrent cough, intermittent fever, pallor, weight-loss and fainting. There is often a family history of a T.B. infection, which occurred many years ago. They are often restless and like to move or travel. The sclera (eye white) often has a bluish tinge. The remedy is also indicated for period problems, nausea, migraine, sweating and a desire for fresh air. (Compare *Pulsatilla).*

Tyler, Sir Henry James. (1827-1908)

The eminent homoeopath born in Mayfair England and father of Margaret Tyler. He was benefactor to the London Homoeopathic Hospital in many generous ways creating the annual Tyler scholarship for studies to the U.S. Many doctors e.g. Weir (see section) were able to take advantage of such scholarships, widening their knowledge to the benefit of homoeopathy.

Tyler, Margaret. M.D. (1857-1943)

Daughter of Sir Henry Tyler, she worked tirelessly for the cause of homoeopathy for over 40 years at the London Homoeopathic Hospital. She was an inspired teacher and lecturer and through the Henry Tyler scholarships, she and her mother, were responsible for the transatlantic links and training of many of our earliest teachers with James Tyler Kent in Chicago. Despite opposition, she gave full support for high-potency prescribing and the single remedy. As a physician she was totally dedicated to her work, patients and students. She was editor of *the journal Homoeopathy* from 1932-42. Author of an important paper on *Drosera,* she also wrote a correspondence course in homoeopathy for doctors unable to attend the lectures and formal courses at the hospital. She was particularly interested in the problem of the mentally handicapped subnormal child.
Major writings include:
1942 *Drug Pictures*

Typhoid disease

In the past homoeopathy has played an important and primary role in the treatment of typhoid. It is now a secondary supportive treatment. Because of the extreme virulence of the disease, it is better to use modern antibiotics when available. The vital energy is often unable to rally when faced with such a severe attack. For completeness, I am listing the major remedies which can benefit the condition.
REMEDIES
Antimonium crud., Arsenicum, Baptisia, Bryonia, Carbo veg., China, Croton tig., Nux vomica, Phosphoric ac.

Typhus Fever

This highly infective tic-born fever is also best dealt with by antibiotics, because of its virulence and danger to the patient, particularly the young, with homoeopathy playing a supportive role in convalescent stages. Again for the sake of completeness only, or where hospital or medical treatment is not immediately available. I am listing some of the principle remedies which may be indicated.

REMEDIES

Agaricus, Arsenicum, Carbo veg., Sulphur.

U

Ulcer - Peptic

One of the commonest diseases of our time. As man increasingly lives in an environment, refined in both ideals and food, cut off from his origins and often family life, isolated from the meaning and end-result of work, insensitive to spiritual values, he pays the penalty in terms of overall general health, especially of the digestive system. Having created a void, he often fills it again with meaningless activities, which usually takes the form of eating, to relieve tension and anxiety. Nature abhors a vacuum, so too does the psyche and it rushes to fill it with fantasy, insecurity and often fear. All of this takes its toll in terms of peace of mind, which is essential for healthy digestion. Acidity, flatulence, burning-pains, hot-air bubbles of wind, burping are common expressions of inner stress and strain. Rushed instant meals are swallowed un-chewed and washed down un-savoured. At other times, phases of over-eating and over-drinking starve the body of vitality in an attempt to survive the excesses. All of this combines to create an 'ulcer climate' with acidity and spasm causing deep pain radiating to the shoulder blades, back or shoulder. A peptic ulcer may cure spontaneously and completely without further symptoms or scar-tissue creates problems of narrowing, blockage and mal-functioning. There is a risk of haemorrhage if an artery in the base of the ulcer becomes eroded. This may produce either the vomiting of fresh blood or its presence in the stools as undigested blood, the stool, black and tarry in appearance. Both are serious and may indicate the need for surgery. A chronic ulcer which has been neglected for many years may eventually become cancerous. Whenever possible, an ulcer should be prevented at an early stage by a reasoned, balanced, rhythmic life-style at all levels and an overall philosophy. When ulceration occurs, it should be treated as early as possible.

REMEDIES

Argentum nit.(bleeding), *Arsenicum, Kali carb., Nux vomica, Ornithogalum, Phosphorus* (bleeding), *Sulphur.*

Ulcer - varicose

The common complication of long-standing varicose veins, usually occurring in the lower leg and associated with obesity or chronic constipation. Ankle oedema and varicose eczema may be present and not infrequently there is a history of recurrent ulceration. A precipitating cause may be a slight trauma to the ankle area. Treatment includes rest, elevation of the limb, and leg exercises to stimulate the circulation. The ulcer should be cleaned with *Calendula* tincture and kept covered with a dry sterile dressing. When infected and discharging pus, cover the ulcerated area with *Calendula* ointment or honey and change the dressing after 3 days. Repeat the procedure until any pus has cleared.

REMEDIES

Calcarea carb., Carbo veg., Causticum, Hamamelis, Lachesis, Merc. sol., Pulsatilla, Sulphur.

Uranium Nitricum (Nitrate of Uranium)

Recommended for diabetic problems where there is an excess of sugar in the urine (glycosuria).

Urethritis

The condition may be gonorrhoeal in origin or non-specific. Diagnosis and differentiation can usually only be made by microscopy of the discharge, which may be thick and creamy yellow. Cystitis is commonly associated with frequency and burning pains. It is usually sexually-transmitted and can become chronic with scar-tissue formation and an intermittent discharge. In gonorrhoeal conditions, a course of Penicillin is recommended followed by the homoeopathic remedy.
REMEDIES
For gonorrhoeal urethritis:- *Medorrhinum, Merc. sol., Sulphur.*
For non-specific urethritis; - *Petroleum, Silicea, Staphysagria.*

Urinary Difficulties

When little urine is passed the cause may be obstructive as in the infant with phimosis, the outlet pin-prick in size and the prepuce balloons-out whenever urine is passed. Treatment is surgical and circumcision. Following surgical intervention, the bladder may lose its power of contraction due to irritation from the operation or anaesthetic. For post-operative retention *Causticum* is the remedy of choice. Slowness or inability to pass urine may be due to nervousness or impossible when another person is present indicates *Natrum mur.* After a stroke there may be paralysis of the bladder nerve supply, and *Opium* is recommended. With prostate problems there is often delay and slowness or a sense of incomplete emptying, requiring *Sabal serr.* For the older woman, the corresponding problem is ‘spotting’ of urine, or slight leaking when rushing, laughing, sneezing

or coughing. This often occurs because of damage to the bladder sphincter muscles during childbirth.
REMEDIES
Causticum or *Sepia.*

Excessive flow and frequency may be nervous in origin or due to infection, sometimes diabetes.
REMEDIES
Argentum nit., Ignatia, Sarsaparilla.

A small renal stone may cause severe colicky or 'sticking' pains.
REMEDIES
Berberis.

Urinary infection is a common condition (See Cystitis).

Urtica Urens (Stinging Nettle)

Tincture of the fresh flowering plant. One of the most ancient remedies with a reputation as a blood purifier. It is useful for scalds and burns, urticaria, rheumatism and for insect bites. Recommended by Compton-Burnett (see section) for gout and as an organ remedy for the spleen. The skin is typically red, irritating or itchy and restlessness is a marked feature.

Urticaria

The acute and often recurrent allergic condition, due to stress or allergy, generalised or local, with several circular patches of raised red wheals on the skin, accompanied by itching and frequently malaise. The urticarial eruption may come on rapidly causing severe anxiety, swelling of the face and throat with malaise.

REMEDIES
Aethusa for allergy to milk.
Astacus for allergy to shellfish.
Fragaria for allergy to strawberries.
Pulsatilla for allergy to pork.
Also consider *Apis, Rhus. tox., Sulphur, Urtica.*

Ustilago (Corn Smut, the maize mushroom)

A uterine remedy for congestive menopausal problems and ulceration of the cervix uteri.

Uterine Problems

Careful examination and correction of any displacement or mal-positioning, must be carried out at an early stage in treatment. Fibroids, either single or multiple, are a common problem (See section).
REMEDIES
Fraxinus, Phosphorus, Silicea, Tarentula hisp.

For flooding associated with the menopause or fibroids.
REMEDIES
Lachesis, Senecio, Sulphur, Ustilago.

For prolapse, usually caused by childbirth.
REMEDIES
Sepia.

Uva Ursi (Bearberry)

Recommended for problems of chronic cystitis.

V

Vaccination

Vaccination is recommended for very virulent infective conditions which can totally annihilate the vital reaction of the individual during an epidemic, or where there is a special risk. Homoeopathy is helpful to ensure that the side-effects of vaccination are minimal. For example, Influenza can be of considerable risk to both the elderly and the very young during an epidemic. In such cases when there is a specific vaccine for the specific epidemic, it should be used. The homoeopathic alternative is the nosode *Influenzium,* which has proved of enormous value in the past when 'flu has reached epidemic proportions. Non-specific vaccination by the 'flu vaccine, unrelated to any specific epidemic, is not generally recommended, as the protection is minimal, unless there is a specific reason to give it (e.g. patients in an institution, or those particularly vulnerable). Typhoid, typhus, or yellow fever, should be treated by a conventional specific vaccination programme where there is exposure and wherever the disease is severe or epidemic. Smallpox is now very rare and virtually eradicated, and in most cases vaccination is not routinely recommended unless there is a special risk, or where the disease is still endemic. Polio vaccine should be given in its conventional form whenever there is any danger of infection. The whooping cough vaccine may carry a considerable risk to the vulnerable child and the specific homoeopathic alternative of *Pertussin* is sometimes recommended as being effective without the danger of a cerebral reaction. Homoeopathy is recommended for the side-effects of conventional vaccination. Use *Thuja* 6 for local problems of pain, swelling, abscess formation, irritation of the skin or fever. Give the remedy three times daily until the condition has cleared and then stop. For conditions of a more general nature, where ill-health dates from a previous vaccination, give *Thuja* in the 30c or 200c potency according to, the degree and severity, of the symptoms. The final decision on vaccination must be an individual one. There are homoeopathic nosodes available as alternatives for all the common diseases and the final decision, whether to conventional vaccination or a homoeopathic nosode, must be a personal one, with an intelligent weighing-up of the virulence of the disease at the time and its incidence, either at home or in a country to be visited. When infection or exposure carries a high risk, then use conventional vaccination, treating side-effects with homoeopathy, unless there are contraindications, when homoeopathy can be used as a first-line prevention.

Vaginismus

Vaginal spasm during the sexual act. The condition is involuntary and nearly always psychological in origin. It is rarely associated with pain or inflammation after childbirth or due to trauma.
REMEDIES
Ignatia, Natrum mur., Platina, Pulsatilla, Staphysagria.

Valerian Officinalis (Valerian)

The important remedy for excitable psychological states with agitation and restlessness, especially hysterical behaviour and spasms of excitability. Pains are changeable and variable, worse for rest and ameliorated by movement (compare *Rhus tox.)*. There is a headache, sore throat, indigestion with nausea, canine hunger, weight loss and diarrhoea. Sighing with tears is frequent, the menstrual pattern painful and irregular. Restlessness at night with increasing agitation and anxiety may prevent sleep.

Varicella (Chicken-pox)

The common infectious disease of childhood. There is an incubation period of about 13-14 days. Diagnosis is by the typical rash with blisters or vesicles followed by pustules and scab formation but without permanent scarring. The rash typically contains at the same time, all three phases of its development. The vesicles are highly infective, and it is still wise to isolate acute cases from the elderly, because of the danger of shingles in this age group. The disease gives a life-long immunity in most cases. Varicella can occasionally occur in the adult when it may pursue a much more severe course with malaise, high fever and prostration lasting for several weeks. Rarely meningitis or encephalitis is a complication.

REMEDIES

Antimonium tart., Merc. sol., Nitric ac., Psorinum, Rhus tox., Sulphur. The specific varicella nosode both prophylactically and during treatment.

Varicose Veins

The common problem of dilation of and tortuosity of the veins of the lower limb. The leg is swollen, the veins irritating with eczema and ulcer formation, in severe or neglected cases. Common causes are:- an increase in circulatory back-pressure from any obstruction or pressure which blocks the flow or weakens the valves and walls of the venous vessels. The commonest cause is chronic constipation, the heavy, overloaded large bowel putting its weight on the long veins of the limbs. Another obvious and frequent cause is pregnancy when the weight of the gravid uterus, causes similar obstruction and back-pressure. Obesity also aggravates the condition. Other reasons for blockage may be the weight of a fibroid, a cyst or other tumour causing mechanical blockage and weakening of the venous walls. Piles is a form of varicose veins, involving the anal-rectal venous area. The causes are basically the same as in other areas. A high fibre diet with extra bran should be taken, whenever there is a problem of constipation.

REMEDIES

Carbo veg., Fluoric ac., Hamamelis, Pulsatilla, Sulphur, Vipera.

Variolinum (Smallpox nosode)

For prevention of the disease when epidemic, and also useful in shingles. The skin is infected with boils, pustules, severe acne and pustules. Also for the scarring of severe or chronic acne (compare *Thiosinaminum).*

Veratrum Album (White Hellebore)

A major remedy for collapse, lifelessness and shock, with extreme chill, pallor and often cyanosis or a mauve-blue tinge to the person. There is profuse sweating, which is drenching and always feeling icy cold. Diarrhoea is frequent and watery as in Cholera. Also for violence, agitation, impulsiveness and restlessness (compare *Tarentula),* puerperal psychosis and suicidal depression. It is valuable after head injury with concussion (compare *Helleborus)*, for headache of a violent pulsating type (compare *Glonoin)* and severe premenstrual tension with irritability.

Veratrum Viride (The White American Hellebore)

For circulatory problems where there is a general congestion or the danger of an impending cerebral attack or stroke (compare *Opium)*.

Vertigo

The common complaint of dizziness due to inner-ear disease and disturbance with nausea and increasing deafness due to degenerative changes. In epilepsy, it may form part of the warning aura of a major attack. With others, it may reflect a minor 'petit mal' attack or part of temporal-lobe irritation. A common cause is hypertension or raised blood-pressure associated with pounding headaches. Often the exact cause is unknown and it reflects an underlying anxiety or stress problem. Careful diagnosis and investigation is always necessary.
REMEDIES
China, Cocculus, Conium, Salicylic ac., Natrum mur., Nux. vomica, Pulsatilla, Spigelia, Sulphur.

Viburnum Opulus (High Cranberry)

The menstrual remedy for dysmenorrhoea, where the flow is of brief duration. Cramping pains occur in the stomach, intestine and uterus. Also for miscarriage of the third month, bleeding, pain at ovulation.

Viburnum Tinus (Lauristinus)

The cardiac or respiratory remedy for oppression in the chest and shortness of breath. The patient holds a hand to the heart in a gesture of weakness and anxiety and the pupils may be irregular.

Vinca Minor (Periwinkle)

The valuable scalp remedy for:- lifeless hair, hair loss, patchy alopecia, an itchy scalp, eczema, skin or scalp infections associated with hypersensitivity of the area and redness.

Viola Tricolor (Pansy)

Recommended for chronic skin condition with infected eczema or impetigo. There is a thick yellow discharge and severe irritation. It is also helpful for enuresis.

Vipera Redi (Viper Venom)

The remedy for severe phlebitis, with venous engorgement and irritation. Also for phlebitis and varicose ulcers.

Viscum Album (Mistletoe)

For lack of vital reaction or collapse. The pulse is slow, the blood-pressure lowered, exhausted and short of breath, on the least movement or exertion. A remedy for the most desperate and extreme conditions. (Compare with *Veratrum alb.*).

Visual Fatigue

Eye strain due to excessive reading or close work, often from poor light conditions and always better for rest. There may be a need for new spectacles, or the ocular lens is unable to focus correctly, from disease or due to age. Cataract is a common cause of visual fatigue. Psychological factors can also play a role.
REMEDIES
Alumina, Calcarea carb., Euphrasia, Gelsemium, Ruta, Zinc. met.

Vital Energy

The inherited vital principle or life force, present throughout life and undermined by disease, miasm or stress. It is the first part of the person affected when disease occurs and this causes the early symptoms of malaise, fatigue and irritability, or lack of interest which precede the development of symptoms - often by several months. Vital force attaches itself in a protective way to the disease process, in order to bind and contain it, protecting the vital organs. The homoeopathic remedies in the higher potencies act first and foremost upon the vital energy reserves, supporting its protective functioning role. It is usually the first area to be relieved by homoeopathy as the remedies act from the centre outwards and according to the homoeopathic law of cure, the more generalised symptoms, such as malaise, jaded indifference, fatigue, lack of energy are relieved first and before other more specific symptoms.

Vomiting

This can be a serious symptom which may or may not be accompanied by nausea. Every case needs careful consideration and investigation of the underlying factors and any surgical conditions excluded. Causes vary considerably, with emotional factors common in children and adolescents (anorexia). In hysterical illness it may be a worrying symptom, often defying diagnosis and treatment. Other common causes are due to a dietary indiscretion, the reason usually obvious and the effects short lasting. Alcoholism is a familiar factor. Other causes include:- peptic ulcer, hiatus hernia, acute infective conditions of childhood and also the central nervous system e.g. meningitis. Blood may be vomited, either fresh blood or mixed with food and partially digested. Bleeding or vomiting from an intestinal obstruction may also require urgent surgery. The problem should be under medical care and if there is doubt, investigations carried out to clarify the underlying causes.

REMEDIES

Aethusa, Arsenicum, Cocculus, Ipecac., Natrum mur., Nux vomica, Phosphorus, Pulsatilla.

W

Warts

The common viral skin infection, occurring on any part of the body with outgrowths of a rough irregular type which may bleed or spread by contact to adjacent skin areas. In general they should not be interfered with and usually there is a good response to homoeopathy. Large warts on the soles of the feet need special attention if enlarging or bleeding and may require surgery. Anal or genital warts with a stem or cauliflower surface, indicate a sycotic miasmic condition and require thorough treatment by the homoeopathic method.
REMEDIES
Antimonium crud., Causticum, Dulcamara, Fluoric ac., Nitric ac. Thuja.

Weir, Sir John. G.C.V.O., M.D. (1879-1971)

The eminent physician and homoeopath to the royal family (The late Prince of Wales, King George VI, Queen Elizabeth the Queen Mother, the present Queen Elizabeth, the present Prince of Wales also Princess Anne, Princess Alice and the Duke of Gloucester) and the late King of Norway. Weir qualified in Glasgow in 1906 and was immediately influenced by Gibson-Miller, who treated a condition of boils, which had not responded to conventional treatments, with such success, that he became his homoeopathic mentor. With the support of Tyler (see section) in 1908 he studied with both Allen and Kent (see sections), at the Chicago Hering Homoeopathic College, returning to become physician to the London Homoeopathic Hospital in 1910 and Compton-Burnett Professor of Materia Medica in

1911. He was an impressive advocate of the single dose and non-interference with any aggravation-response by the patient. President of the Faculty in 1923, his lectures, addresses and articles were numerous, with a directness and simplicity which is refreshing. In spite of his eminence, Weir was always regarded as a man of enormous humility.

Wells, Phineus Parkhurst. M.D. (1808 - 1891)

The 19th century homoeopathic physician from Brooklyn, New York, who became the first President of the International Hahnemannian Association (1881). He was co-editor of the *American Homoeopathic Review.*

Wesselhoef, Conrad. M.D. (1834-1904)

The American homoeopath, active in the last half of the 19th century.
Major writings include;
1872 The cause of contention between the old and the new
1880 The method of our work
1881 A plea for a standard of the attenuated dosage
1883 Is the homoeopathy of Hahnemann the homoeopathy of today?
1883 The law of the similars
1887 How to study the materia medica
Also translator of Hahnemann's *Organon* in 1876.

Wheeler, Charles Edwin. M.D. (1868-1946)

The Australian homoeopath, who trained at St. Bartholomew's and was staff member of the London Homoeopathic Hospital from 1904. President of the

British Homoeopathic Society and the International League, he was a stimulating writer and lecturer.
Major writings include;
Introduction to the Principles and Practice of Homoeopathy
Fools or Knaves - a defence of homoeopathy
Chronic Diseases (written with E. Bach)
He was also involved in a translation of the *Organon.*

Woods, Harold Fergie. M.D. (1883-1961)

The homoeopath who was a student of Kent in Chicago with Weir on a Tyler scholarship in 1908. He returned to support the case for high potency prescribing and the single dosage. Physician at the early Children's Homoeopathic Dispensary in Shepherd's Bush, founded by Robertson Day in 1920 and later amalgamated with the London Homoeopathic Hospital in 1935. Consultant to the London Hospital, he was a founder member of the International League in 1925. In spite of increasing blindness he remained an active exponent of homoeopathy, a gifted prescriber and physician.
Major writings include:
The Essentials of Homoeopathic Prescribing
Homoeopathy in the Nursery
Herbal Simples

Whooping Cough

A highly infectious condition of infancy and childhood marked by attacks of paroxysmal coughing leading to blueness of the face, as the larynx and respiratory muscles go into spasm, followed by a long, deep breath causing the characteristic whoop - which is diagnostic. Paroxysms of coughing lead to vomiting or congestion, with nose bleeds. The condition may last weeks and often follows a drawn-out course. It is mainly of danger to the very young child, but in recent years the illness has largely followed a milder pattern.

REMEDIES

Pertussin prophylactically from six months, unless there has been a direct contact, when it can be given earlier. The nosode may need to be repeated every six months until the age of five. During the acute illness give *Pertussin,* and consider *Arnica, Ant. tart., Belladonna, Carbo veg., Drosera, Ipecac., Nux vomica, Phosphorus.*

Worms

These occur as Round Worm (Ascarides), Threadworm (Oxyuris), Tapeworm (Taenia). Of these, by far the commonest is the threadworm. See separate sections.

Wounds

In all cases stop the bleeding by local pressure, or a tourniquet applied intermittently. Shock must be treated by keeping the patient warm and giving *Arnica* or *Veratrum alb.* If more severe, repeat *Arnica* every few minutes until there is a response. Careful cleaning of the area is essential when hospitalisation is not considered necessary, or is unavailable. All foreign matter must be removed and the wound cleaned with *Calendula* tincture. When large, or in a cosmetic area, suturing should be carried out. A clean sterile dressing must be applied over the *Calendula.* Tetanus vaccination is required for a dirty wound. When in doubt the patient should be taken to the nearest hospital casualty department, homoeopathy acting as an additional supportive therapy to conventional treatments.

REMEDIES
Aconitum for restlessness and agitation.
Arnica for shock.
Arsenicum for infection.
China for loss of blood.
Hypericum for nerve damage and shooting pains.
Ledum for punctured wounds.
Phosphorus for persistent bleeding.
Veratrum alb. for collapse.

Wright-Hubbard, Elizabeth. M.D. (1896-1967)

The New York born graduate of Columbia and one of the first women graduates to specialise in homoeopathy working in New York for most of her life. She was editor of *The Journal of the American Institute of Homoeopathy* and first woman President of the American Institute of Homoeopathy, also President of the International Homoeopathic Association 1945/46.
Major writings include:-
A Brief Study Course in Homoeopathy.

Wyethia Helenoides (Poison Weed)

Recommended for severe chronic dry cough, hay fever and pharyngitis.

XYZ

X-Ray (Ethanol exposed to x-ray)

For any conditions, particularly of the skin, but also of any organ of the body which has never functioned well since exposure to x-ray diagnosis or radiotherapy treatment. It is a useful remedy for cancer treatment, also for alopoecia and pain or discomfort after an x-ray examination.

Zincum Metallicum (Zinc)

One of Hahnemann's major anti-psora remedies for chronic conditions of agitation and restlessness with nervous twitching or convulsions. The condition typically involves the lower limbs and feet with 'fidgety feet', and oversensitivity to the least noise of stimulus. Its neurological sphere of action includes paralysis and meningitis.

OTHER INSIGHT PUBLICATIONS

The Side-Effects Book
Dr Trevor Smith

This book describes in detail the most common hazards of our pressurised society, the props used and their risk to health. It is of interest and value, to both patient and doctor alike.

For those who wish to extend their knowledge of a particular field, the list of references and further reading is invaluable.

Chapters include:- The Developmental Stages of life, Stress and the Home, Sexuality, Over-The-Counter Drugs, Health Products and Vitamins, Medically Prescribed Drugs, Surgical and Cosmetic Procedures, Immunisation, Food and Diet, Social Addictions, Holidays and the Sun, Travel, Sport, Occupations, Animals and Plants, Household Products, Pesticides, Drugs of Dependence and Misuse, Pollution.

'One can only marvel at the breadth and scope of this work' - Homoeopathy Today

'The Medical Mrs Beeton' - Hampshire Chronicle

'A book about giving people more basic information' - Today Newspaper

Understanding Homoeopathy

Dr Trevor Smith

The revised second edition of this popular book. It is an comprehensive introduction to the homoeopathic method, explaining the basic principles of homoeopathy in clear, simple terms, which can be readily understood by the beginner.

Topics discussed include:- What is Homoeopathy, The Basic Causation of Disease, The Indications for Homoeopathy, Advantages of the Homoeopathic Approach, Preparation of the Remedies, Homoeopathy and the Home, First-Aid Remedies.

The author also discusses the approach, indications, choice of remedies for the most common health problems of the family, and when the they should be used.

Talking About Homoeopathy

Dr Trevor Smith

This book is taken from a series of talks and lectures, given over several years, and forms an invaluable reference book for anyone wishing to have a deeper knowledge of homoeopathy.

The author is a practising homoeopath, and writes clearly about a variety of topics of general interest which offer a deeper understanding and a more challenging awareness of homoeopathy, its indications, potential, and scope of action.

Chapters include:- Emotional Problems and how the homoeopathic approach can be used to resolve them, The Nature of Illness, Remedies for the Homoeopathic Medicine Chest, The Difficulties of Self-Prescribing, Insomnia, Tension, Holiday Remedies, Homoeopathic Potency, The Homoeopathic Nosodes, The Science of Individualization, The Gentle Kitten.

The Principles, Art and Practice of Homoeopathy

Dr Trevor Smith

A book which explains in simple language the principles of homoeopathic practice and prescribing.

It includes chapters on :- Dosage, Potency, First and Second Prescriptions, Homoeopathic History Taking, the Consultation, the Principles of Homoeopathy, Symptoms and the Patient, The Positive Value of Symptoms, The Homoeopathic Constitution, Modalities, 'Proving' a Remedy, Miasms, Temperament, Vital Energy, Prognosis and Prediction in Homoeopathy.

A second section is concerned with Constitutional Prescribing and the role of homoeopathy in the treatment of Cancer.

A final practical section, shows how best to work out your own 'Constitutional' and gives reference sheets for the major constitutional profiles.

Emotional Health

Dr Trevor Smith

A major study of the causes and remedies for emotional health problems. The author is a holistic doctor, psychiatrist, and also a homoeopath.

The books represents a comprehensive up-to-date survey of the most common emotional problems facing people living in the twentieth century. It identifies these problems and then explains the best, practical self-help steps that can be taken to solve them.

Simple guidelines are given in order to promote healthier attitudes, changes in specific problem areas, and better psychological perspectives.

Topics covered include:- Security, Shyness, Relationships, Mood Swings, Coping with Divorce, Depression, Nervous Breakdown, Preventing Breakdown and Strain, Building Health Ego Strengths.
Fear and modern Man, Psychology and Everyday Life, Emotional Tension, The Importance of Relaxation, Visualisation, Chronic Emotional Problems, Physical Health and Psychological Balance.

Personal Growth and Creativity
Dr Trevor Smith

This book describes in detail the most effective ways to stimulate and develop personal creativity and growth, in order to bring about positive changes in outlook.

The book offers practical guidelines that will lead to constructive results. Within a short space of time, you learn to identify both the physical and psychological obstructions to creative development and discover how to remove these obstacles and open the doors to greater personal growth, achievement and happiness.

Topics include:- Physical Blocks to Creativity, Social and Environmental Blocks, Psychological Blocks to Growth, Creative Workshops, Overcoming Blocks to Creativity, Attitudes that Develop Creative Potential, Exercises to Expand Creativity.

Homoeopathy for Pregnancy and Nursing Mothers

A comprehensive self-help guide to the common problems which may occur during pregnancy, at birth and during the early months of motherhood.

Homoeopathy for Babies and Children

A comprehensive self-help guide to the homoeopathic treatment of the everyday health problems the modern mother has to cope with.

Homoeopathy for Everyday Stress Problems

A comprehensive self-help guide to the common stress problems of our modern pressurised society.

Homoeopathy for Teenager Problems

A comprehensive self-help guide to the most common problems of adolescents and how to understand and treat them using homoeopathy.

Homoeopathy for the Menopause

A comprehensive self-help guide to the emotional and physical problems of the menopausal woman, to help revitalise health and energy.

Homoeopathy for Psychological Illness

A comprehensive self-help guide to common psychological illness problems which, often cause misunderstanding, alienation and unhappiness.